The Menopause
Guide

The Menopause Guide

Danna Demetre, R.N.

SPIRE

So many people influence our lives. Some meet us for a season and make a meaningful deposit in our souls. Others journey with us for a lifetime and never cease to be a source of strength and wisdom. There is one special woman who has been there for me and modeled grace and love every day of my life. She always told me that pregnancy and childbirth were "no big deal," menopause just another "phase" of life, and even breast cancer was a mere "speed bump." I dedicate this book to the wisest, most loving woman I know, Mary Lou Shansby. I want to be just like you when I "grow up," Mom.

Contents

Contents

Acknowledgments

I've been blessed to have professional and ministry partners that are also among my dearest friends. What a blessing to have our professional and personal lives intersect in such significant ways. There are three people in particular who have journeyed with me, supported me, prayed for me, loved me, and sharpened me in deep and meaningful ways. First, I want to thank my husband of twenty years, Lew, who has described his calling in part as being the "man behind the woman." It takes a big man to make a statement like that. He's the guy who runs alongside, gives me incredible encouragement, and picks up the pieces when I've pushed myself beyond my limits. Second, a huge hug and thank you to Terri Podlenski. She was my first lifestyle client, then my business partner, and ultimately the best girlfriend I've ever known. She's my editor, cheerleader, prayer partner, "reality checker," business administrator, promoter, chief financial officer, and reliable confidant. Last, I have deep gratitude that God chose to sharpen me in so many ways through my radio partner, adopted big brother, and last but not least, pastor, Dr. Tim Scott. He has taught me how to think biblically, apply spiritual truth accurately, and maintain a sense of humor and hopefully grace in the process. My life is richer, my ministry is fuller, and my heart is transformed because of you three. And thanks above all to Jesus Christ, who provides the way to continue these incredible journeys together in eternity.

Preface

Walk a Mile in My Pumps

Shoulder to shoulder, hip to hip,
We'll get through it together if we don't quit.

Purse to purse and pump to pump,
We'll hurdle the hurdles and jump the jumps.

Head to head and heart to heart,
I'll show you the way; I'll help you start.

Faith to faith with Christ as our head;
We'll get through this life by the blood he has shed.

I'll show you the way over life's big humps;
Come along, my friend . . . walk a mile in my
    pumps.

—Danna Demetre and Diana Twadell

Not long ago, menopause was considered the beginning of
old age, and women only whispered to each other about going

through "The Change." Now, menopause is a family affair. It was estimated in the year 2000 that over 50 percent of American women entered some phase of menopause. Today, four thousand women in the United States and Canada enter menopause daily! (Talk about global warming!) We're the largest unorganized club out there. Perhaps with a little synergy, we can change the world. We certainly have enough "heat" to make some kind of impact!

The sad truth is, most women don't celebrate this phase of life. Our culture worships youth and perfect bodies. We look in the mirror and find one more wrinkle, gray hair, or "liver" spot (I absolutely hate that description) every day. We don't feel like we did in our thirties. We don't look like we did in our thirties either. And some days, we don't even think like we did yesterday.

Can you relate?

"*Why* am I in this room?" I know I'm not alone. Come on; admit it. You've asked yourself this question more than once. You know how it goes. You walk into a room for a specific purpose, but by the time you get there, you can't for the life of you remember *why* you're there. When I was younger, I called these mental "dead air" moments brain freezes. Today, I simply call them "meno-pauses." Wouldn't it be great if these frustrating occurrences came with a recorded message that played spontaneously, warning those nearby with this announcement: "This is a test of the menopause brain freeze system . . . This is only a test . . . Should this brain freeze occur for more than a few seconds, please reset the system by administering chocolate or caffeine."

According to Christian psychologist Dr. Maryann Rosenthal:

Menopause is a new and natural phase of life affecting women between the ages of 40 to 55 years of age and beyond. Perimenopause is the stage before periods cease completely and can begin as early as our mid-thirties. This is the best time to lay the foundation for good health in later years. There is an overwhelming amount of information about menopause and yet, women still feel ill prepared and misinformed. We all must become proactive and be our own advocates when it comes to both the physical and psychological changes that come with this new and important passage in our lives. After all, we will be in menopause until the day we die, and we need to develop our own personal plan. I think that we overlook the fact that menopause involves not just the ovaries and the uterus, but also the brain. Eighty-five percent (85%) of women will experience menopausal symptoms, both physical and psychological; some of these symptoms will go away and some will not.[1]

The ability to cope with the changes of menopause depends upon:

- Genetic heritage (How did mom, grandma, and auntie cope?)
- Emotional and spiritual outlook
- Attitude
- Support
- Outside stressors in your physical environment and your life[2]

So how about you? Are hot flashes, PMS, fatigue, low libido, memory loss, or night sweats getting you down? I've "been there, done that!" However, I'm here to tell you that there is life not only after menopause but in its midst. In fact, I am *certain* that the best years you will ever experience are yet to come *if* you have the right perspective and *if* you take good care of yourself.

13

9-2-10

That's what this book is all about—taking care of you from the inside out . . . body, soul, and spirit. Many of the chapters relate directly to menopause, but I've included others simply to help you embrace and celebrate this very special season of life. While I believe the ability to laugh at ourselves is essential, I have interwoven some deep spiritual truths and serious topics through these pages. I've gone to God's Word to find the principles and truths that are timeless even though our physical bodies are not. I pray that each chapter will entertain, inspire, and teach you how to maximize the most important time of your life . . . now!

Health Flashes for Holy Hotties

I sure hope you're not offended by being called a "holy hottie." But that is what you are, isn't it? A godly woman with hot flashes! You are still a sexual, complete woman until the day you die, despite your declining hormones and increasing wrinkles. The better you take care of your aging body, the better you'll feel and the more fully you'll embrace life.

From mood swings to burning belly fat, I will address a variety of health topics at the end of each chapter to help you enhance your vitality and wellness for decades to come. I will also devote several full chapters to issues such as hormone replacement therapy, lifestyle nutrition, and nondiet approaches to permanent weight loss.

Despite my experience as a registered nurse and health reporter on my weekly radio show, I don't intend this book to be a complete resource for addressing all the physical challenges of menopause and aging. I've teamed up with many of my Christian health professionals to address the very real physical challenges and health concerns mature women face including, but not limited to, our laundry list of menopausal symptoms.

My good friend and naturopathic physician, Dr. Mark Stengler, is quoted frequently throughout the book. After you read about healthy concepts related to many aspects of our journey toward ultimate "maturity," you may desire more in-depth information from sources such as Mark's book *Your Menopause, Your Menotype*.

There is also much to be said about weight loss. If you struggle with diet and eating issues, I recommend my book *Scale Down: A Realistic Guide to Balancing Body, Soul and Spirit*.[3] I have listed many other excellent resources in Recommended Resources at the end of this book.

It's Your Body

I hold to the philosophy that we are ultimately responsible for our own self-care. We are the CEOs of our health-care team. Let's hire and fire wisely! While we cannot be an expert in all areas, we must be well informed. Whether our objective is weight loss or menopause management, the essentials never change.

It's time for a major health alert! If you don't begin to make changes now, your body may never bounce back. This season of life can be your most rewarding. But if your health is compromised by poor habits, you cannot possibly live it to the max! This is the season where you are most vulnerable to disease. How you live will impact your life span profoundly. The good news is that aging can be a new motivator to finally "do the right things for the right reasons." In reality, most of you *know* many things you can and *should* do to improve your health. The challenge is more often figuring out how to consistently implement those healthy changes. Lack of time is always an issue. But don't forget that not taking the time to care for your body will potentially rob you of some of the most important years of your life.

God has given us incredible resources to live fully in each season of life. It seems women centuries ago didn't have near the challenges we do today in getting through this phase of life. On a physical basis, much of that has to do with our lifestyles, but on a mental and spiritual basis, it has to do with our attitude. I hope you will find *The Menopause Guide* a wonderful blend of humor, hope, and healthy solutions that will heat up your joy and maximize the best years of your life!

"Sistering" through the Seasons of Life

My dear friend Pam Farrel is an international speaker and author of many books who has loved and mentored more women than any other woman I know. She often uses a building term called "sistering" that describes how carpenters nail two boards together in places such as doorways to create a strong and unshakeable framework. When we "sister" other women, we come alongside them and make them stronger by our physical, mental, emotional, and spiritual support. I want to thank all the women in my life and those who were transparent enough to share their menopause journeys in this book. Your sistering has made me wiser and stronger, and your stories will help others build an unshakeable foundation for not just surviving but thriving during menopause and beyond!

Medical Disclaimer

This is a reference book based on research by the author, and the ideas and suggestions in it are not intended as a substitute for the medical advice of your personal health professional. All matters regarding your health require medical supervision. Consult your physician before adopting suggestions in this book as well as about any condition that may require diagnosis or medical attention. Statements made by the author regarding certain products and services represent the opinions of the author alone and do not constitute a recommendation or endorsement by the publisher. The author and publisher disclaim any liability arising directly or indirectly from the use of the book or any products mentioned herein.

1

The Three Ps of Womanhood

As I see it, all women who live long enough will go through three phases of womanhood: Puberty, Pregnancy, and "Plasticality" (a.k.a. ready for plastic surgery). Obviously, every one of us must pass through puberty. Some women will never experience pregnancy either by choice or by circumstance; nevertheless, their bodies are designed for its "potentiality" with all the physical and emotional manifestations. And if we live long enough, most of us will at least feel as if we could use a little plastic surgery whether we choose to have it or not!

Phase One: Puberty

It seems God starts preparing women at a very early age for maneuvering the speed bumps of life. In order to fulfill the roles he calls us to, we need to go through a type of "hormonal boot camp" to be fully ready for all life may dish out. And this hormone roller coaster is not only a conditioning exercise for adolescent girls, it is payback time for moms! You remember all the times *your* mom said, "Just wait until you're in my shoes!" Those of us who are "blessed" with teenagers soon realize that they are "payback" for the years when we were teenagers! Enjoy.

Do you remember the transition from carefree little girl to womanhood? One day you were running around the playground like a little tomboy and the next thing you knew, you were encumbered with pads, tampons, and an odd feeling that some simplicities of childhood were gone . . . forever. Or at least for another twenty-five or thirty years!

They broke the "good news" to us in our fifth grade health education class. We were briefed about our impending metamorphosis with cutting-edge film strips explaining that one day very soon we'd become women. But the actual "event" hit like lightning, and the next thing I knew was that I *didn't know* this strange new person living in *my* body! *Where did these monthly mood swings and cramps come from? Is God punishing me for something?* I remember sitting in the bathroom in seventh grade thinking, *This isn't fair. I didn't sign up for this.* I felt weird, awkward, and cranky. I still do.

Phase Two: Pregnancy

We eventually got over the initial shock and resigned ourselves to "it"; "the curse"; "that time of the month"; or "the cycle." Then, we were at least partially prepared for the next phase—pregnancy. I don't know about you, but I had all sorts of idealist notions of how perfect it would be. I'm sure a few too many movies and not enough pregnant friends led to those winsome thoughts. I didn't get much time to reconsider. One month off the pill and—voila—mission accomplished! Early morning nausea burst my optimistic bubble the first month. The subsequent body morph was next.

The thing I wasn't ready for was the immediate change in my breasts. Most girls dream of having large breasts. Mine had always been average. But for the first time in my life, I had compassion for Dolly Parton. It was really frustrating when part of my body entered a room a few seconds before I did. I'm sure most people thought I'd had plastic surgery. I wanted to wear a sign reading "Under temporary construction" or "Don't look here; I am not an object."

Then, at about eight months, my belly button popped out! How disgusting. I was a labor and delivery nurse, and I thought I'd seen everything. But it looked a whole lot different when it was my body staring back in the mirror. Having a baby is a full-body experience, a total act of sacrifice. I didn't know that my sweet baby was the ultimate parasite. My twenty-something daughters are still gaining frequent nutrition, not from my body but from my wallet!

Once you've huffed, puffed, and pushed that baby out, you think your body is your own again. But, no; now you've converted from incubator to refrigerator. Or, as comedian Paul Reiser puts it from a man's point of view, you've turned your entertainment center into a refreshment stand. Breastfeeding is the most awesome experience. God in his wisdom allows *you* to create your baby's perfect food. Wow. Nevertheless, there are times you want to scream like a two-year-old while holding your engorged breasts, "Mine! These are mine!"

Well, girlfriends, as they say, we've "been there and done that!" I hope this has been a nice reminder of those challenges we left behind. Now we move forward. If we have a healthy perspective, it could be the best phase of all.

Phase Three: Plastic Surgery

Whether you've experienced pregnancy or not, something starts to happen somewhere between the ages of thirty-five and forty-five: the realities of time, gravity, and relaxation kick in. Everything that was up is now going down. And everything that was tight is getting loose, except perhaps your favorite jeans. Your breasts fall a little, your buttocks sag, your skin wrinkles, and you even start to get shorter! You've now entered

---

I think this story that was shared via email with an anonymous writer says it all:

THE LOVE DRESS

A mother-in-law unexpectedly dropped in on her new daughter-in-law. She rang the doorbell and opened the unlocked door. Stepping inside, she found her daughter-in-law standing naked near the entrance, eyes wide open in shock and surprise at her unexpected intruder.

"What are you *doing*?" the mother-in-law asked.

"I'm waiting for my husband to come home from work," the daughter-in-law answered.

"But you're NAKED!" the mother-in-law exclaimed.

"This is my Love Dress," the daughter-in-law explained sheepishly.

"Love Dress? But you're naked!"

"My husband loves me to wear this dress! It makes him happy and it makes me happy. I would appreciate it if you would leave now because he will be home from work any minute."

The mother-in-law was tired of all this romantic talk and left. On the way home she thought about the Love Dress. When she got home she got undressed, showered, put on her best perfume, and waited by the front door. Finally her husband got home. He walked in and saw her standing naked by the door.

"What are you doing?" he exclaimed.

"This is my Love Dress," she replied.

"Needs ironing," he said.

---

the "plastic zone." You are officially ▓▓▓ of ▓ ▓al candidate for plastic surgery.

About the time our lives make sense and we know "who we are," our bodies decide to go on vacation. The one thing we could look forward to—getting rid of our period—is replaced by hot flashes, memory lapses, and a new kind of mood swing.

It just isn't fair. Do you ever feel like there is a conspiracy against your body coming at you from all fronts? Well, the poor woman who wrote the memo below sure believes it's true. She decided to email all her friends and sound the warning bells. I never found out who she was, but I think I might have experienced the same thief! This is what she wrote:

My thighs were stolen from me during the night of August 3rd a few years ago. It was just that quick. I went to sleep in my body and woke up with someone else's thighs. The new ones had the texture of cooked oatmeal. Who would have done such a cruel thing to legs that had been wholly, if imperfectly, mine for years? Whose thighs were these? What happened to mine? I spent the entire summer looking for them. I searched, in vain, at pools and beaches, anywhere I might find female limbs exposed. I became obsessed. I had nightmares filled with cellulite and flesh that turns to bumps in the night.

Finally, hurt and angry, I resigned myself to living out my life in jeans and Sheer Energy pantyhose. Then, just when my guard was down, the thieves struck again. My rear end was next. I knew it was the same gang, because they took pains to match my new rear end (although badly attached at least three inches lower than the original) to the thighs they had stuck me with earlier. Now my rear complemented my legs, lump for lump. Frantic, I prayed that long skirts would stay in fashion.

Two years ago I realized my arms had been switched. One morning while fixing my hair, I watched, horrified but fascinated, as the flesh ▲ upper arms swung to and fro with the motion of the ha... ...n. This was really getting scary. My body was being replaced, cleverly and fiendishly, one section at a time. In the end, in deepening despair, I gave up my T-shirts. What could they do to me next? Age? Age had nothing to do with it. Age was supposed to creep up, unnoticed and intangible, something like maturity. NO, I was being attacked, repeatedly and without warning.

That's why I've decided to share my story. I can't take on the medical profession by myself. Women of America, wake up and smell the coffee. That isn't really "plastic" those surgeons are using. You know where they're getting those replacement parts, don't you? The next time you suspect someone has had a face "lifted," look again! Was it lifted from you? Check out those tummy tucks and buttocks raisings. Look familiar? Are those your eyelids on that movie star? I think I finally may have found my thighs . . . and I hope that Cindy Crawford paid a really good price for them!

This is NOT a hoax! This is happening to women in every town, every night . . . Warn your friends!!!!!!!

The "Stuff" That Matters Most

There's lots of "stuff" in life that we have to deal with. The three Ps of a woman's life are unique to our feminine journey. Some of us will have greater challenges than others. Extreme menstrual pain, difficult pregnancies, or the loss of an un-born child can stretch us to our limit. The journey through menopause has its own distinctive path for each woman as well. Roller-coaster hormones often result in roller-coaster emotions. These emotions can dramatically skew our ability to stand on the truths we know because we may feel out of control, on the edge, or at the end of our rope. We must not give in to those lies. Truth is still truth whether we "feel" it or not.

I love what James says in chapter 1, verses 2–3: "Consider it all joy, my brethren, when you encounter various trials, knowing that the testing of your faith produces endurance." He goes on to tell us that we must "let" endurance have its perfect result, so that we may be perfect, lacking in nothing. I'm not sure how I am perfected in getting through the "trials" of menopause, but I do know it has surely tested my husband's endurance.

Often, when I deal with common life challenges like this, I wonder why God has allowed us to go through these difficult phases. I think we must continually remind ourselves that since man rebelled in the garden, things are not and will not be according to God's original design. Don't forget, part of the curse was aimed directly at us in Genesis 3:16. To the woman, he said, "I will greatly multiply your pain in childbirth, in pain you will bring forth children; Yet your desire will be for your husband, and he will rule over you." It's not supposed to be easy anymore! So, if childbirth is difficult, why not the journey out of those years?

Whether our trials are external in the form of circumstances or internal in the form of bodily changes, we can take them and grow in faith and endurance. The constant reminder of our "humanness" reminds us that the very best is yet to come. It forces us to run to God whether for more patience or more forgiveness as we negotiate these raging waters called menopause. We need to remember to do the things we *know*, not the things we *feel* in this time of transition. This is what we know:

1. We need to pray as if prayer is the very air we breathe.

2. We need to worship the Lord, experiencing his refreshing Living Water.
3. We need to nourish our minds with the truth of his Word.
4. We need to digest these truths through quiet meditation.

Little meaningful change and few worthwhile objectives can be accomplished apart from God. Sure, we can go through all sorts of exercises in self-improvement, but any external change leaves us only temporarily satisfied. I'm not making a legalistic statement on plastic surgery, hormone therapy, or even good nutrition. But the truth is that all those things are secondary to the condition of our souls and spirits. If those are nourished daily, we will be just fine no matter what hormones or life may deliver. Yes, God is even in control of hormones. So, stop for just a moment and do what you know:

- Send up a quick prayer; give God both the essential and the trivial aspects of your day. He knows what's going on. Talk to him. Express your concerns. Pray for wisdom. Surrender your stuff.

- Worship God for who he is right here, right now. He inhabits your praises; tell him how you feel about him. Don't keep reading. I'm *serious*. Now is a great time to praise and worship the One who loves you above all others, so much so that he has engraved you in the palms of his hands!

- What one verse truly feeds your soul in this season of your life? Write it on a card. If you don't have a favorite verse, find one. It's there, waiting to be discovered. (And don't do that "let the Bible fall open" thing. You could get something like "for there is nothing good for man under the sun except to eat, to drink and be merry.")

Study, pray, and read. You will find the right verse in the course of your study. And, when you do, memorize it and fully digest its truths. God's Word is living and active. Let it do its work in you.

- Spend some quiet time in meditation before this day is done. It may have to be in the car or shower. That's okay. God's presence is a balm to your frazzled mind and your weary soul. Don't procrastinate. Just do it!

All that being said, I do think that many of the ordeals of menopause can be vastly minimized by simply living more healthfully. By that I mean eating as close to what God originally intended, managing our stress, and getting sufficient sleep and exercise. We intensify our symptoms by our unhealthy lifestyles. So, while menopause is "natural," all the negative symptoms may not be. When you look back in time, women didn't always complain of the intensity of symptoms we have today. (And I just will not believe that our sisters of old were simply not complainers, will you?) In fact, in Asian cultures the women don't even have a word for PMS or hot flashes because they don't experience those kinds of reactions. Why? Most experts believe their diets and lifestyles are the significant factor.

HEALTH FLASH
TIPS FOR HOLY HOTTIES

Help for Hot Flashes

You've heard of chicken soup for the soul. Well, we holy hotties need something with a little more punch to deal with those tiresome, sometimes downright annoying, even sleep-

27

depriving . . . hot flashes. But don't run to your doctor for a prescription for estrogen just yet. Give a few natural remedies a try first. I'll discuss more about hormone replacement therapy—the good, the bad, and the ugly—later. If you've already tried some natural remedies and didn't get sufficient relief, it is very likely that you were not taking enough to create a therapeutic benefit. I tried several before getting the result I needed. You will note recommended dosages below.

As my radio cohost, friend, and personal naturopathic physician Dr. Mark Stengler always says, "It's better to start with the simplest, most natural approach first and see if it helps before moving on to more expensive and elaborate measures." Even though he is very comfortable with natural hormone therapy, he believes that less than a third of women need it. And those who do rarely need to stay on it indefinitely. For now, let's consider some affordable and less extreme approaches to our symptoms.

Black Cohosh

The leading herbal treatment in Europe for women suffering from "hot flashes" is black cohosh. More than forty years of research have noted that this herb contains specific compounds called triterpene glycosides. They have estrogen-like activity and help with estrogen balancing. To get the best results, Dr. Stengler recommends a dosage of 80 to 160 milligrams per day depending upon the severity of symptoms. Some women may need to take these higher doses both morning and night until symptoms abate.

Vitex

Vitex is another herb that can help to support the pituitary gland, which is responsible for estrogen and progesterone production. It is thought to be an "adaptogenic" herb, which means it helps provide a balancing effect on the female hormonal system from puberty through menopause. It is best used on a long-term basis, with most women noticing improvements within two to four months. Caution: Vitex should not be taken by women taking birth control.

Formulas

There are many menopause formulas on the market that are very effective in diminishing many of the symptoms of menopause. The one that has been most effective for me was actually formulated by Dr. Stengler. It's called Liquid Menopause Formula by Innovative Naturals. The liquid doesn't have the greatest taste, but I am currently living without any menopause symptoms! In fact, I think I might be getting younger!

Don't expect these natural supplements to work like an aspirin when you have a headache. They generally need to be taken for several weeks (and sometimes even months) to get the full beneficial effect. In the meantime, have patience, pray for cool weather, and put a fan in your bedroom!

Taking Action

Most people read a book and get inspired in the moment but never implement what they learn into the details of life. If you take some time *right now* to reflect on this chapter, chances are you'll be stimulated to think, pray, and implement the changes you desire. If you simply read and never take personal action, nothing happens.

Take a few moments to briefly answer the following questions. Then transfer onto an index card the important thoughts, ideas, or actions you plan to take. When you've finished the book, you'll need to prioritize your action plan and implement two or three things at a time. If you commit to doing one new thing a week for the next year, you'll be amazed at the new and vibrant woman you'll be living with for the rest of your life!

1. What was the most important truth you gained from this chapter?
2. What changes, if any, do you desire to make related to that truth?
3. What specific thoughts or actions need to be implemented to make those changes?
4. What are your greatest stumbling blocks toward this change?
5. On a scale from one to ten (with ten being the highest) how important is this relative to other needs/changes in your life? Use this scale to help you create an overall action plan when you finish reading this book.

2

What's Wrong with This Picture?

Getting ready every day seems like such a waste of time. Showering, shampooing, and shaving our legs consumes precious hours, not to mention drying, brushing, styling, flossing, and dressing. Phew . . . I'm frustrated just thinking about it. If God had simply made forty-eight-hour days, we'd cut our "beauty regime" investment in half! I guess my "high maintenance" upkeep wasn't a priority on his agenda when he created twenty-four-hour cycles. Oh well.

As I get older, I've found that I can get ready much faster than in years past. I realized that it takes me as much time as I choose to give myself. If I schedule too much, I fritter it away primping and checking out my new "age flaws" in the mirror. I've also discovered creative ways to multitask during my daily routine. Little things like brushing my teeth with one hand and drying my hair with the other. Or doing my sit-ups while my deodorant dries so I can get dressed without getting those ugly white marks on my sweater. These days I only give myself about thirty-five minutes and am generally satisfied with the results. That is, until recently. My streamlined approach backfired on me last Sunday.

Menopause Moments

Getting ready for church is always a challenge. For some reason, Sunday is the one day my thirty-five-minute plan tends to fail me. Something always pops up that robs a few minutes from my well-scheduled routine. Last week I realized I was signed up for Sunday school treats.

These kinds of disruptions call for even more creative multi-tasking methods. I decided to dress while I made a quick call to see if my husband (who left early to work out at the gym) would stop and pick up some goodies on his way to church. He didn't answer. Bummer. I tried on two pairs of black sandals to determine which would look best with my outfit. The phone rang . . . YES! He got the message, and I had recaptured ten minutes. Amazingly, I was out the door on time and arrived with minutes to spare. Walking down the stairs toward our Sunday school class, I noticed my nice pedicure popping out from my sandals. My sandals! Good grief; I was wearing two different shoes.

Was it poor time management or another menopause moment? The latter, I fear. I had to decide quickly how to manage *this* moment with grace. Hmmm. My husband was across the room setting out the goodies. As I approached, I asked him coyly, "Darling, notice anything a little different about me?"

"You covered your gray?" he replied insensitively.

"No."

"A new outfit?"

"You've seen this one a dozen times. Look down."

He noticed nothing! But my girlfriend who was standing close by watching our exchange broke out laughing and called *her* husband over, who joined her in chorus. "We're not laugh-

---

I received an email from a woman who described her experience this way:

I think I have A.A.A.D.D.—Age Activated Attention Deficit Disorder! This is how it goes: I decide to wash the car. I start toward the garage and notice the mail on the table. OK, I'm going to wash the car, but first I'm going to go through the mail.

I set the car keys down on the desk, discard the junk mail and I notice that the trash can is full. OK, I'll just put the bills on my desk and take the trash out. But since I'm going to be near the mailbox anyway, I'll pay these few bills first.

Now, where is my checkbook? Oops, there's only one check left. My extra checks are in my desk. Oh, there's the Coke I was drinking. I'm going to look for those checks. But first I need to put my Coke farther away from the computer. Oh, maybe I'll pop it into the fridge to keep it cold for a while.

I head towards the kitchen and my flowers catch my eye; they need some water. I set the Coke on the counter and, uh-oh! There are my glasses. I was looking for them all morning! I'd better put them away first. I fill a container with water and head for the flower pots—Aaaaaagh! Someone left the TV remote in the kitchen. We'll never think to look in the kitchen tonight when we want to watch television, so I'd better put it back in the family room where it belongs.

I splash some water into the pots and onto the floor; I throw the remote onto a soft cushion on the sofa and I head back down the hall trying to figure out what it was I was going to do.

End of day: The car isn't washed, the bills are unpaid, the Coke is sitting on the kitchen counter, the flowers are half watered, the checkbook still only has one check in it, and I can't seem to find my car keys! When I try to figure out why nothing got done today, I'm baffled, because I KNOW I WAS BUSY ALL DAY LONG!!! I realize this is a serious condition, and I'll get help, BUT FIRST I think I'll check my email.

---

ing *at* you, Danna; we're laughing *with* you!" he exclaimed.
The three of them proceeded to share with everyone entering
class my fashion faux pas.

Later, as we pulled our chair into circles for a group dis-
cussion, I noticed a few latecomers staring inquisitively at
my feet. I had to chuckle. Managing menopause moments
with grace is so much easier when you can laugh at yourself
and let others join in the fun. *However*, I was a little scared
yesterday when halfway through the day I realized I was
wearing two different earrings!

I felt a little better when my ministry partner, Terri, who is ten
years my junior, confessed her own recent brain lapse. One day
as she was driving on the freeway on her way to a very important
appointment, she realized she was still wearing her slippers! Far
from menopause, Terri is thirty weeks pregnant with her first
child. I guess this problem really is a "hormone thing." I really
believe God must enjoy our regular comedy acts.

My friend Kris Peterson tops the list of embarrassing moments. Like most of us, she finds grocery shopping drudgery, so
she tends to move efficiently through the aisles, accomplishing
her chore in record time. One time, however, she was genuinely
delighted that she had collected so many items more quickly
than usual. It wasn't until she got all the way home and began
unpacking the grocery bags that she realized more than half of
what she had purchased was from someone else's list.

Like many of us, she had inadvertently started down the aisle
with a stranger's cart. Most of us would realize it right away
and timidly sneak the cart back without getting caught. Not
Kris. Though she didn't get caught, she unloaded the foreign
items onto the belt for the checker and actually paid for them
without even noticing. Now, *that's* a menopause moment!

Kris could have kept the whole incident a complete secret.
No one would have known . . . *if* she hadn't told a whole room

full of women when she was speaking at our ministry event. Being a veteran "menopauser," Kris has mastered the art of laughing at herself and was compelled to pass on the blessing of a good chuckle to others. I hope you will do the same with your awkward menopause moments.

As I visited various menopause-related websites, I found story after story of women who experienced hilarious menopause moments and were willing to share them with the world. Like Dee Adams, cartoonist and creator of the "Minnie Pauz" card line, says, "One loses many laughs by not laughing at oneself." Here are a few of my favorite stories; don't be afraid to share yours as well!

"Never Mind!"

After reporting to the police that my car had been stolen, I went to rent a car so I could get to work that following morning. On my way back from the place, what did I spot but my forlorn little car, sitting in front of the beauty parlor. I had left it there and walked home for the exercise instead of driving . . . duh. Then later at home when I needed my car to run an errand, it was nowhere to be found. Just imagine my horror when I realized what I had done. I'm still shocked. The worst part was calling the police back and having to tell them, "Never mind!"

Your Place or Mine?

I was spending the day with a new friend. As we were driving back home that evening she said, "You need to turn here." When I asked why, she answered, "Because I live here!" Well, I thought I was taking her back to my place so I was heading in that direction. The only problem with *my* plan was that I was heading to a home I hadn't lived in for two years! All turned out well. I eventually got back to where I really live.

Serial Menopause Madness

On Monday I went to my exercise club with two different aerobic shoes on. On Tuesday I forgot it was Halloween and had to go to the store and buy candies at the last minute. On Wednesday I forgot my dentist appointment. On Thursday I forgot to go to my women's group. On Friday I forgot which car I was driving. On Saturday, in Bible study, I forgot a word that was on the tip of my tongue. On Sunday I forgot to do the laundry. Why can I never forget to eat?

Time Changes Everything

After a week of out-of-town guests, I woke up at 6:30 feeling rested and ready to start the new week with gusto! I fixed my first cup of coffee for the morning and turned on the computer and the television. But, instead of the usual morning shows, there was a football game on one station and a movie on another . . . very strange for a Monday morning! Then I noticed the date on my computer. It said "Sunday, Nov. 25." I immediately changed it to "Monday, Nov. 26" and made a mental note to ask someone what could cause the date to not change on my computer. Then *60 Minutes* came on TV and it finally hit me that the time was 6:30 Sunday evening instead of 6:30 Monday morning, and I had just awoken from an afternoon nap and lost all sense of time.

Please Refrigerate After Opening

Not too long ago, I reached into the pantry to get the flour canister and discovered a half-gallon container of curdled milk that had been there for who knows how long! I felt really badly remembering how I had yelled at my husband for using up all the milk and not replacing it when I wanted to eat cereal one morning. Asking forgiveness is becoming a daily habit!

Don't Swallow

Before applying hand lotion, I took off my wedding ring and put it in my mouth to avoid dulling the diamonds with lotion "scum." I reached for the lotion bottle and was dismayed to see my wedding ring missing from my finger! I looked all over the chest of drawers, on the floor, and even went into the bathroom before discovering, there it was, right in my mouth where I had put it seconds before!

Do you wonder what is going on in your brain as your hormones fluctuate and your moods swing to and fro? There are some powerful things you can do to enhance your mental acuity at any age. As you will learn in the Health Flash that follows, everything that positively impacts your brain will improve your skin as well. Follow those tips and you won't be looking for those keys or showing up in mismatched shoes too often. But, when you do, have a good laugh and share the story. Laughter is the best medicine of all.

HEALTH FLASH
Tips for Holy Hotties

The Brain/Beauty Connection

If you knew there was a powerful nutrient that would stimulate your brain, revitalize your skin, slow down aging, improve fat metabolism, lubricate your joints, decrease inflammation, *and* protect your heart, wouldn't you make sure your body got plenty of it? But what if this nutrient was found in only a handful of foods that you rarely ate on a daily basis? And what if the foods you *were* eating regularly were throwing off a key balance, causing you more damage because you lacked this key nutrient? If you don't address this almost universal nutritional gap, your body and, most important, your brain will be short-changed.

The nutrient I am talking about is an essential fatty acid called omega-3. It is one of only two fats that are considered essential for life, the other being omega-6. Our body cannot produce these fats and must have them to function properly. In addition to the list of great benefits above, I've listed some other compelling facts later in this book. I've been notching up my omegas for about a year and I can see the difference in my skin. And except for my occasional hormonal "menopause brain freezes" my ability to concentrate and recall information is terrific!

Are You Getting Enough Omega-3?

The best sources of omega-3 essential fatty acids are salmon, swordfish, tuna, shark, pecans, almonds, walnuts, soy nuts, flaxseed, and deep-green vegetables like bok choy, kale, and turnip greens. We need the equivalent amount of omega-3 fats we find in a serving of salmon (about 3,500 milligrams) *every* day. All the other sources (even fish) are at least one quarter the amount found in salmon specifically. And we are being cautioned to watch our intake of large fishes because they contain higher amounts of mercury (another sad example of man's lack of stewardship for the resources God has so abundantly provided).

In his *New York Times* runaway best seller, *The Wrinkle Cure*, world-renowned dermatologist Dr. Nicolas Perricone established and documented the incredible benefits of omega-3 fats. He writes that for the quickest nonsurgical face-lift possible, we should eat salmon at least ten times a week! Now if you love salmon, have an unlimited budget, *and* like to cook fish on a daily basis, that might work for you.[1] For the rest of us, there's a much easier, more affordable, and even lower calorie way to get all the benefits—supplementation. Since not all supplements are equal and omega-3 fats can spoil quickly, I did some research and recommend the Ultimate Omegas by Nordic Naturals.

According to naturopathic doctor Jordan Rubin in his book *Patient Heal Thyself,* "There may not be a single nutritional supplement or pharmacological drug today that can offer the same level of protection against cancer, heart disease and the inflammatory response that impacts many other diseases."[2]

The Problem Is, We're out of Balance

The balance of the two essential fatty acids (omega-3 and omega-6) is critical to good health. Omega-6 fatty acids are found in vegetable oils. They are very easy to get into our diets on a daily basis because the food industry made a massive shift away from using animal fats, such as butter and lard, to making products out of vegetable fats. Commercial baked goods, salad dressings, and cooking oils such as soybean, canola, and olive oil are all based on these plant source fats. Yes, they are much better for us than the alternative. But you *can* get too much of a good thing. And almost everyone has.

As a result of this shift, most people probably obtain sufficient omega-6 fatty acids, but our diet is woefully short of the omega-3 fatty acid, creating a huge disparity. This imbalance causes an inflammatory response all over our bodies, hardening areas of the brain, creating cardiovascular disease, decreasing lubrication in our joints, aging our skin, and more. Yuck!

While the ideal ratio of omega-3 to omega-6 should be somewhere between 1:1 and 1:3, the majority of Americans are at ratios of 1:20 to 1:30. Yikes! This huge discrepancy is causing huge health concerns. Since we get sufficient omega-6 fatty acids in our diet, the practical challenge is to eat more of the omega-3 fatty acids. With that in mind, here are a few facts that may motivate you to get your omega-3 intake up ... up ... up!

Fact: Brain and skin are made up of the same type of tissue.

Fact: Anything we do that helps our brain will help our skin.

Fact: The skin is the largest organ of the body.

Fact: The brain is the most important organ of the body.

Fact: Poor lifestyle and diet, ongoing stress, smoking, and environmental pollutants all damage fragile brain cells and damage our skin cells, causing wrinkles and premature aging.

Fact: People who abuse their bodies through poor diet and lifestyle can experience, as early as their thirties, mental fall-off, including mood swings and depression.

Solution: Nourish your brain and enhance your beauty with the powerful ultimate omegas!

Younger Inside and Out

Because brain cells are largely composed of fat, the right kinds of fat in the diet are one of the most critical elements in creating and maintaining brain health. The skin requires the exact same nutrients to stay young or even reverse the signs of aging. The omega-3 fatty acids are the single most important nutrient that feeds our brain and skin.

Many compelling studies are revealing that omega-3 supplementation decreases aggressive behavior, diminishes depression, protects against Alzheimer's disease, and fosters mental clarity. Just imagine your brain as healthy, well nourished, and firing on all eight cylinders, as opposed to under-nourished like a car in bad need of a tune-up and needing a jump start to perform simple tasks. (That jump start would be coffee and sugar, perhaps?)

The same goes for your skin. With good omega-3 nutrition, it's healthy and well nourished. Each cell is plumped up like a ripe grape, smooth and firm, instead of shriveled up like a raisin. We can spend a fortune on creams and makeup, but nothing takes the place of skin care from the inside out!

Are you motivated to make the brain/beauty connection? Pick up some salmon and walnuts today at the store, invest in a quality omega-3 supplement, and you'll be looking, thinking, and feeling your best!

Taking Action

1. What was the most important truth you gained from this chapter?
2. What changes, if any, do you desire to make related to that truth?
3. What specific thoughts or actions need to be implemented to make those changes?
4. What are your greatest stumbling blocks toward this change?
5. On a scale from one to ten (with ten being the highest) how important is this relative to other needs/changes in your life? Use this scale to help you create an overall action plan when you finish reading this book.

3

Mirror, Mirror . . . Please Lie!

We've already acknowledged that we've entered the third "P" of life—the stage where we seriously consider various options that will lift, tighten, and enhance specific areas of our aging "bods." So, how do you feel about making it to this unique season? Do you like the woman you see when you look in the mirror? For me, it depends upon what time of day I look! I certainly see a nicer reflection after a little makeup and hairstyling. Nevertheless, I don't think I've ever thought, "Now that's perfection; I finally look just right!" It's just not as important to me as it used to be. How about you?

To the end, most of us will still be just a little concerned about our beauty. I know of women who have instructed their loved ones on what they want to wear and how they want their makeup applied on the day of their funeral! Hey, gals, you're not even going to be there; get over it! I can say that without judgment since I was completely obsessed with my appearance as a young woman.

When I'm feeling like I'm falling back into old, unhealthy thinking about my appearance, one Scripture I try to remember is 1 Samuel 16:7: "For man looks at the outward appearance, but the LORD looks at the heart." Wouldn't it be wonderful if we humans were like God in this area?

For the first twenty-eight years of my life, I hated how I looked. My legs were never lean enough, my hair never right, my skin, teeth, even fingers fell short of the image I desired.

AGING GRACEFULLY

I found a gray hair today which wouldn't be so bad
Except it makes 51 with the ones I already had.
I have wrinkles on my cheeks and dimples on my thighs,
Moles that sprout a hair or two and bags beneath my eyes.

My waist is getting thicker and my teeth aren't quite as white
So, I tell my spouse it's sexier to make love without the light.
I can't remember birthdays or what my kids just said.
It's a miracle that every day I still get out of bed!

But, I have friends around who love me. My husband's my best friend.
God has been so good to me and is with me to the end.
My kids have turned out pretty good. I like my mom and dad.
The joyful days outnumber any that are bad.

I've learned to be more loving, and when to take a stand;
Times that I just listen and when to lend a hand.
I'm thankful for my days on earth however long they be
And hope that in many ways I'm aging gracefully.

And when my days are over and I enter heaven's door
Please, dear God, be full of grace and make me a size four!

Maria Rote

It is incredibly futile and frustrating to be totally discontent with who you are. And often extreme criticism of our outward appearance is simply a deeper criticism of who we believe we are inside *and* out. Ah, the power of perspective. Unfortunately for me, it took many years of emotional pain and yo-yo dieting before I could see myself accurately.

By God's grace, I overcame my sixteen-year struggle with bulimia and emotional eating and learned how to maintain a reasonably lean body *without* dieting! I share my journey to lasting victory in my book *Scale Down: A Realistic Guide to Balancing Body, Soul, and Spirit*. And that victory certainly helped me improve my self-concept. But most important, I learned to celebrate with gratitude the body and appearance God chose to give me.

Now, even though I've been quite content with my body for the last two decades, I have to accept the fact that this "earthly tent" is starting to give in to gravity. Turning fifty was a humbling experience! I must remember that one day all who have a saving faith in Christ will have absolutely perfect glorified bodies. Hallelujah.

My Body . . . My "Self"?

In today's culture, how we look seems to have more significance than who we are. We are bombarded with magazine and television ads that tell us we need to look a certain way. Those ads influenced me profoundly thirty years ago. I can still remember a cigarette commercial that exclaimed, "You can never be too thin or too rich." Sadly, Karen Carpenter, a pop singer of the late sixties and early seventies, believed that lie. She didn't live long enough to overcome it, but her untimely death resulting from complications from a prolonged eating disorder screamed out to the world, "Your lies are killing us!"

Today, the pressure is even greater. Beauty and our dispro-
portionate attention to seeking the current "look" is really a
matter of focus. One of the best things we can do to develop
healthy body images is change our focus. As it is said, "Beauty
is in the eye of the beholder." We must avoid the constant messages that influence how we perceive ourselves if we want to
celebrate with gratitude who we really are. That being said,
where should Christians draw the line when it comes to addressing beauty and appearance?

This is such a difficult issue, because of the social stigma.
We allow the straightening of teeth through orthodontia and
the coloring of hair when age brings a certain gray tone.
There is a touch of hypocrisy in some who will not allow
plastic surgery under the notion that all plastic surgery is
selfish. If a child is born with a cleft palate, we certainly
allow for surgery to fix not only the palate but also the vis-
ible deformity of the cleft lip often accompanying a cleft
palate. The logic seems to be that if it is a birth defect, then
it is justifiable. However, someone's intense insecurities
about appearance can be emotionally disabling. Ideally, we
should accept God's sovereignty and accept our shortcom-
ings physically or aesthetically.

All plastic surgery is not equal. For example, what of the
case of a woman who survives breast cancer and has had a
radical mastectomy? The reconstruction is about appearance,
her sense of femininity, and probably many other important
factors. This surgery certainly would not be denied by the
judgmental moralist, or would it?

What of the case of a man who has been in an accident and
has a facial deformity—would this be considered legitimate?
In the case of a woman who was obese for years and has lost
a vast amount of weight—should she be allowed to have a
tummy tuck to remove extra skin?

My recommendation for those who consider plastic surgery is make sure you go into the process realizing that you are the same person before and after the surgery. God loves you and so do your friends, regardless of the flaws you may be stressing about. You will probably be insecure after the surgery. My recommendation for those judging others who have plastic surgery is: stop! Love your brother and sister even when you disagree. Romans 14:2–4 says

> One man has faith that he may eat all things, but he who is weak eats vegetables *only*. The one who eats is not to regard with contempt the one who does not eat, and the one who does not eat is not to judge the one who eats, for God has accepted him. Who are you to judge the servant of another? To his own master he stands or falls; and he will stand, for the Lord is able to make him stand.

So does plastic surgery dishonor God as creator? This cannot be answered fairly in sweeping generalities. It is probably true that some plastic surgery procedures are an insult to the creative act of God. However, we should allow God to judge this for others. In regard to yourself, if you struggle with this view, avoid the surgery.

How Do You Really See Yourself?

What do you see when you look in the mirror? Oftentimes, no matter how much weight we lose or how many changes we make to our outward appearance, we still are unhappy with the image reflected in the mirror. This unhealthy body image is the result of unhealthy thinking. It takes years of unhealthy messages to develop these negative body images. And it will take consistent, healthy, affirming truths to erase and replace them! Like me, many women see themselves inaccurately.

When our perception of our body image is off, we find it difficult to let go of what we think we should look like and celebrate and accept what God designed us to be. This is not to say that we shouldn't desire a leaner or more toned body or want to dress in fashion and wear makeup. But the key is to do the right things that promote reasonable results and accept the results with gratitude. How do we do that? As I explain in detail in my book *Scale Down*, we must erase and replace all of our lies about not only how we look but also our habits by renewing our mind with truth.

Looking at the Right Reflection

Building a healthy body image requires an accurate perspective of who we are inside and out. Romans 12:2 states that we are to be "transformed by the renewing of our minds." That transformation comes from knowing and believing that God sees us as beautiful, acceptable, and desirable despite the world's unrealistic values. That means we must see ourselves correctly and change the messages in our minds about what is beautiful. Our current culture may tell us that tall and very thin is the ideal body type. But when we look at all of the women in our lives, we see that most don't fit that mold. Do you want to conform to the world's image or embrace the wonderful creation you are?

There is incredible freedom in celebrating with joy exactly who you are today! To do so, you must decide to invest time and energy in thinking differently. Look around you. How many of the people you see every day look perfect by today's standards? Not many. Just imagine if you did not pick up one magazine, newspaper, or catalog in the next five years. What if you never watched one minute of television? What would your physical expectations of yourself be? Accepting and celebrating your body and appearance would be much easier if you stopped comparing them to an unrealistic standard.

Christ-Confidence

We don't want to be simply "self-confident" and accept our flaws. I think the ultimate goal of a mature Christian woman is moving beyond self-confidence to Christ-confidence. We can gain an incredible personal contentment when we learn to see ourselves through our Creator's eyes.

Take an inventory of your current attitudes and identify your unhealthy thoughts. Surrender them to God. Ask him to help you discard those lies you believe and fully embrace the truth of who you are in Christ—physically, emotionally, intellectually, and spiritually.

Are you able to actually thank God for who you are? Do your thoughts about yourself glorify God? I will dig into these important principles in more depth in a later chapter.

For now, just try to refocus your attention on seeing yourself from God's viewpoint. He sees you as a complete person—body, soul, and spirit—and is most concerned about who you are inside. I suggest you pray that he gives you a clear perspective and grateful spirit not only for who you are potentially but also exactly who you are this very moment.

In addition to praying for an accurate perspective, it is very important that you reverse your negative thoughts by telling yourself the truth. For example:

- "God created me and I am always beautiful in his eyes."
- "With God's help, I can have a healthy and reasonably lean body."
- "I celebrate my body and realize it is not the sum of who I am."

- "I can enjoy life without always thinking about how I look."
- "I am focusing on my strengths more than my perceived flaws."

Remember this: you are a unique person with incredible value. You have your own set of strengths and weaknesses. Some people may be a bit closer to their potential, but that does not diminish your worth in God's eyes. A healthy body image is not one that allows you to see yourself as better than others but rather celebrates with thanksgiving what God has given you.

No matter how hard we try or how great we may appear to the world, we are all imperfect creatures. Yet, each of us was created for a purpose with unique talents and potential.

A Lifelong Battle with Truth

Researchers tell us over and over that "beautiful people" get more attention. Statistics reveal that those who are seen as attractive by current norms are more likely to acquire better jobs, higher pay, and a host of other privileges "average" people don't receive. It's not fair, but that's how the world responds. However, *you* don't have to conform to this unreasonable standard regarding outward appearance. With God's help, you can change your perspective. As I said before, it's a matter of focus.

Perhaps God has given you beauty according to the world's standard. Perhaps he didn't. Whether he did or not, remember that we are all blessed in a variety of ways with both human attributes and spiritual gifts. One person is not better than another. We are all equal in God's sight. Our human perspectives have changed our perception of what is valuable.

Finding a Balance

I want to encourage you to find a healthy balance. Let's propose to make lifestyle changes that ensure a healthier body tomorrow with a celebration of who we are today. That will help us live each day to the fullest. I love Psalm 118:24, which says, "This is the day which the LORD has made; let us rejoice and be glad in it." We need to learn to live in the moment and celebrate the gifts God has given us to the fullest, realizing that we never completely "arrive" in any area of life, this side of heaven.

In the lifestyle classes I teach all over the country, I remind women that our bodies are the only vehicles we have to get around in this temporal life. Too often we choose the expedient lifestyle change that helps us lose weight quickly or overcome some other physical challenge without regard to the ultimate effect it will have on our health. This is my personal motto: <u>Do the right things for the right reasons and leave the results up to God</u>.

Spiritual Exercise

I encourage you to let God work through you to produce whatever results he pleases. Trust him to give you a satisfaction that penetrates your heart to your very soul. As you surrender your current body image to God, ask him to help you identify the lies you believe. When you replace the lies with truths from God's Word you will be amazed at the transformation that takes place. It is so important to block the unhealthy images from television, movies, or magazines and become deluged with images of how God sees you. Your perspective of your own beauty will change dramatically. Spend time each day in the arms of your heavenly Father, asking him to help you see yourself accurately. Surrender your insecurities and frustrations to him. Choose to walk in the confidence of who you are in Christ—a truly beautiful woman from the inside out!

HEALTH FLASH
TIPS FOR HOLY HOTTIES

Extreme Makeovers

When surveyed, most women will say that the areas of their life that most need changing are diet and exercise. We also know that no matter what happens to the economy, the cosmetic industry is rarely impacted in a very negative way. Women care about their looks. This is not news to anyone. On one end of the spectrum are those who make beauty their life's obsession. On the other end, those who have given up on beauty say they don't care and relegate themselves to sweat suits and ponytails sans makeup. I'm guessing most of you probably fall somewhere in the middle. You care but are not obsessed about your appearance. Those who care most get a little discouraged as the gray hairs increase, the waistline expands, the buttocks sag, and the face droops. Watching ourselves age is difficult for some.

Attractive people get more attention than those who are homely; this is a sad reality. I've been watching the contestants on ABC's *Extreme Makeover* shows with fascination. There is no doubt that these people's lives are being changed profoundly just by changing their looks. As I watch the contestants return to their spouses and families, I pray that all the changes are for the good. Will the changed outward appearance change who they are at their core?

Do you ever wonder what God thinks about our efforts to stay young and look beautiful? I do. Is it acceptable to wear makeup and color our hair but is it going too far if we submit to Botox injections or a full face-lift? Many wonderful treatments these days are relatively inexpensive and deal with fine lines and sagging skin. Does a godly woman's pursuit of beauty diminish her spiritually? I don't know if there are any hard and fast rules to these questions. I do believe that what I've already said about gaining Christ-confidence and having an accurate identity is our foundation, no matter where our beauty quest may take us.

True Confession

Before I turned fifty, the only cosmetic treatments I had were occasional glycolic facials. I learned that these procedures naturally stimulated collagen growth and diminished wrinkles. But, at age fifty, I began to hate the fine lines around my mouth. So, I decided to explore collagen injections. In the process, I met a wonderful Christian cosmetic dermatologist, Dr. Peter Rullan. He shared how medical technology, skin care, and nutritional supplements have advanced so rapidly that most women who take good care of themselves will never need surgical face-lifts. I proceeded to have more intense glycolic treatments by Dr. Rullan and had him do small injections of collagen around my lips. They look full and smooth like they did when I was thirty. Is that a bad thing? I don't think so. But, if I couldn't afford that treatment, I think I could handle having a few extra wrinkles.

Since then, Dr. Rullan has removed a few small moles and done a laser treatment to smooth the skin on my neck and chest. With all this amazing, almost pain-free technology, it is easy to see how women can spend thousands of dollars pursuing a youthful appearance. I began to understand why some go too far and become walking billboards for why not to have plastic surgery. I had to take an inventory of my personal convictions and boundaries and decide not only what fit into my budget but what I felt right about pursuing from a beauty perspective. I asked myself this question: "If money or technology were not available, could I celebrate my beauty and age with as much passion?" I truly believe the answer is yes. I hope I'm not deceiving myself.

The Healthy Way

One thing I know for sure is that taking care of ourselves will slow down aging more than any procedure or surgery ever can. Eating right, exercising, and stopping bad habits such as smoking or excessive drinking are essential. I am amazed at how much better my skin looks since I've increased my intake of fish oil and eaten more healthfully. Of course, exercise is great for circulation and promotes an excellent complexion. We know what to do; we just need to do it!

The Natural Way

At seventy-four, my mother is a very attractive woman. She dresses stylishly and applies her makeup well. She is full of life and has a great smile. She hasn't colored her hair for years, nor has she ever had any cosmetic surgery. In fact, at age fifty-six, she had a complete mastectomy and never opted for reconstructive surgery. She has been a great model of balance for me. Her comfort with her body image is inspiring.

How we pursue beauty is a very personal issue that we each need to grapple with on our own. If we think our value is somehow increased because we look more youthful, we are mistaken. But, if a little procedure here and there gives a lift (no pun intended), I say . . . go for it. For me, I'd prefer to see a mature woman with the natural character a few wrinkles bring than the "ponytail too tight" look so many women are wearing today in the quest to be forever young.

Let me reemphasize what I've already stated before: when Jesus returns in his glory, we will all receive our perfect, glorified bodies that will never decay. Now that's something to look forward to with great joy!

Taking Action

1. What was the most important truth you gained from this chapter?
2. What changes, if any, do you desire to make related to that truth?
3. What specific thoughts or actions need to be implemented to make those changes?
4. What are your greatest stumbling blocks toward this change?
5. On a scale from one to ten (with ten being the highest) how important is this relative to other needs/changes in your life? Use this scale to help you create an overall action plan when you finish reading this book.

4

The "Change" That Transforms Your Life

Ladies, we're more than halfway through our lives, and despite our tenure on this planet, almost every mature woman I've met has a personal speed bump that trips her up. Maybe for you, it's an unhealthy relationship with food or a deep sense of insecurity. Possibly you struggle with panic attacks, persistent negative emotions, or just wish you weren't such a procrastinator. Perhaps you've read many books on the subject of your concern or been involved in an accountability group but still keep hitting the same brick walls. You can read all the spiritually grounded self-help books on the market and never change one aspect of your life if you don't get to the root of all change—your mind.

As you read further in this book about your changing body and perspectives on living this season of life with great passion and purpose, you need to know that all change you desire to implement must start first in the recesses of your mind.

God designed your mind to be the pilot of your soul. If your thoughts are inaccurate or unhealthy, your emotions and behavior will be as well.

A Transformed Woman

I met an attractive woman named Carol about seven years ago. Though she was quite overweight at the time, the first thing I noticed was her beautiful face and radiating smile. What I learned about Carol saddened me deeply. She shared that her husband of decades would not come near her physically; he told her frequently how repulsive she was to him. Because we believe what we are told most often, Carol came to believe she was an ugly, worthless woman.

She decided to take my lifestyle weight management class to lose weight in hopes her husband would find her attractive. Carol did lose weight, but the most important change happened between her ears. She came to celebrate who she was with or without extra fat on her body, without the approval of her husband. Despite Carol's transformed mind and body, her husband still chose to leave. Carol stood confidently on the "rock" of her salvation. One of her favorite tools from my class was a scriptural self-talk tape that helped her see herself accurately and celebrate her true identity in Christ. She still listens to that tape! Seven years later, she's a voluptuous, radiant, and self-confident woman. Carol recently sent me an email with a desire to encourage other women who have struggled to be "good enough":

Soon I'll be 55. Robert, my grandson, says "that's old." I guess that's true from a fourteen-year-old boy's perspective. My son-in-law, Patrick, has a more positive outlook. He told me, "Soon you'll be a 'Double Nickel.'" I guess in his culture that's "hot." Wow, I'm a Double Nickel . . . I'm finally a "Perfect 10" (like Bo Derek through the backdoor). There is another side of this "Double Nickel" life—I just don't sweat the small stuff anymore. Today everything that used to be astronomical is now small stuff. For example, my perspective about my weight has changed dramatically. I've stopped hating being a "full-figured" woman. Learning that Marilyn Monroe was a size 14 and still considered one of the sexiest women to live has helped me change my self-perception. I don't have to fit in with today's standard of beauty. So, today at 55, I'm happy with my healthy and shapely body. It is so true that "we are what we think"! I have experienced that a renewed heart and mind brings forth a renewed body, soul, and spirit. Ah yes, how I praise God for the renewed mind that compels me to do the right things for the right reasons. I love the "Double Nickel" life!

You Are What You Think

The renewed mind . . . it is a life-changing reality for anyone who is willing to do the simple yet time-consuming work of identifying your lies and replacing them with transforming truth. From bad attitudes to destructive beliefs, your mind is the pilot of all your soul. It compels all your emotions and behaviors. What you feel and all your actions are based on what you truly believe. If you struggle with self-discipline, negative attitudes, or significant insecurities, change your behavior and feelings by first changing your mind.

This is a powerful truth that can change your life for the better or for worse. Through repeated input, we will ultimately become programmed to see ourselves according to our most dominant thoughts, ideas, and experiences. If you *think* you are out of control with food or unable to change, the truth is . . . you probably are! If you say you hate exercise, you prob-

57

ably do. If you think you always fail, you probably will. <u>Be careful what you allow to enter your mind on a daily basis. In essence, what goes in will come out.</u>

Getting in Tune with Self-Talk

What do you say when you talk to yourself? Perhaps you are not even aware that you are talking to yourself. But we all do. Pay a little closer attention throughout the day to the things you are saying in your mind or even when you speak about yourself to others.

How do you describe your body, your fitness, your energy, your self-control? If you keep telling yourself negative thoughts, you'll continue to believe them. And those negative beliefs will sabotage your ability to make lasting, positive change. <u>Remind yourself frequently that you believe what you tell yourself most often. That is why your behavior often feels out of control.</u>

One of my favorite verses is Romans 12:2. It says, "Do <u>not be conformed to this world, but be transformed by the renewing of your mind." *Transformed.*</u> I love that word. If our mind drives all of our emotions and behavior, we must learn to act on this profound truth.

There is nothing complicated, magical, or mystical about changing our minds. God designed our brains so that they will respond to the most dominant messages. If yours are lies, then change them with truth. Many verses in the Bible address the importance of our minds and how we think. God's prescription for renewing our minds is clearly communicated in Paul's letter to the Philippians. He outlines what we must do. Here's what Paul wrote:

> Whatever is true, whatever is noble, whatever is right, whatever is pure, whatever is lovely, whatever is admirable—if any-

thing is excellent or praiseworthy—think about such things. Whatever you have learned or received or heard from me or seen in me—put it into practice. And the God of peace will be with you.

Philippians 4:8–9 NIV

Underline the four words "think about such things." This illustrates in part what renewing our mind is all about. It's about dwelling on "the right things" consistently. Amazingly, we can witness actual physical changes in the brain's neuron pathways as we change the frequency of certain messages. They will actually grow or shrink depending on how often they are activated in our mind. These physical changes take many weeks or months to become discernable in our conscious thoughts, feelings, and resulting behavior. But, over time, the result is profound.

And just as important, there is incredible power in God's Word. In fact, this is what the apostle Paul says about that power:

The word of God is living and active and sharper than any two-edged sword, and piercing as far as the division of soul and spirit, of both joints and marrow, and able to judge the thoughts and intentions of the heart.

Hebrews 4:12

According to the Bible, God's Word actually divides our soul and spirit! And that sharp, two-edged sword is not some long-wielding blade used against our enemy. In this case, it is a short, surgical-type knife that we turn on ourselves. Yes, when we turn the truth of God's Word on ourselves, it will divide the truth from the lies. In fact, his Word will help us judge the thoughts and intentions of our hearts and change our minds. A changed mind will ultimately change our life.

I have applied this profound spiritual truth to my life over the decades. After five years of counseling without any significant relief, I found incredible victory from debilitating panic attacks. Similarly, my battle with bulimia was slowly won after more than fifteen years of out-of-control bingeing and purging. I am not negating the benefits that a quality, biblical therapist can bring to the process of dynamic change. However, I know there are numerous people who are totally renewed by feeding truth appropriately and consistently to their minds over and over. Therapists agree that ultimate change occurs when lies are identified and then erased and replaced with dynamic truth.

Did you ever hear the phrase, "It takes twenty-one days to change a habit"? That's because the neuron pathways in your brain don't even begin to change until you've told yourself a new truth and practiced a new habit for at least that long. The reality is that the longer you practice a new behavior, the easier it becomes. Therefore, you must exercise a certain level of personal discipline before you actually sense any internal changes. Whatever you do repetitively will become locked in. You are the steward of your mind. Be very careful with what you think, say, or do on a regular basis.

Without even thinking, we revert to that which we've done most often, sometimes to our own dismay. We all demonstrate the power of repetition in the things we seem to do by automatic pilot. I remember once when I got a new car with an emergency hand brake after driving for years with a foot break. For a couple weeks, I tried to set the foot brake that was no longer there every time I parked my car! Without conscious and deliberate effort, our minds will revert to the strongest programs. If some of the programs are unhealthy or ungodly, we need to change them before they become autopilot behaviors and attitudes in our lives.

The first and best place to go for truth that will transform our lives is God's Word. We can also take many practical steps to transform our thinking and ultimately change our behavior by addressing the thoughts and attitudes that are tripping us up.

One of the most effective ways to change our thinking is to get in tune with our "self-talk." That is not some kind of New Age technique for self-actualization. We all talk to ourselves. Unfortunately, most of us aren't paying attention to what we are really saying in the privacy of our own minds. That's a mistake. Those silent, ongoing conversations are a huge part of our autopilot programming, and that self-talk can be changed.

As I shared in my book *Scale Down*, these truths are known and accepted by the biblical teachers and psychologists all over the world. For example, in his book *The Healing Power of the Christian Mind*, Dr. William Backus comments on the subject of self-talk:

> As a clinical psychologist and pastor, I've been aware for decades how dark depressive thoughts and negative self-talk create more emotional problems than the actual events that trigger our emotions. Self-talk refers to the way we mentally process events—that is, how we interpret things that happen to us. That's why it's important to understand how our self-talk—those statements we make to ourselves—form our emotions: powerful feelings like fear, anger or worry.
>
> Today, I am convinced that strengthening your spirit with bold, encouraging, life-giving truths that are revealed in the Bible—God's Word—will help you move toward physical wholeness and overall well-being. The Spirit communicates with your mind and your mind communicates with your body. The truth has a positive impact on our bodies when it is be-

lieved and when it is allowed to change our state of heart—that is, our moods and character.[1]

We don't seem to have any trouble feeding our minds all sorts of mental "junk food." What is so hard about putting good information into our brains? Nothing. We just don't do it. The steps to change our thinking and ultimately our behavior are quite basic. Sadly, very few people master this discipline. I believe that's because our society expects—even demands—quick-fix solutions to almost every challenge. Changing our minds requires a consistent, daily supply of powerful messages. We are personally responsible to take control and ensure the regular delivery of those messages. If we don't choose to purposely infuse transforming truth into our minds, we are surrendering control to our old lies or the negative influence of the world.

There is also a huge difference between knowing something and truly believing it. As Backus says,

> You can identify certain foods and "believe" they exist and in fact can nourish you, but they do not until you eat them. Like real food, truthful ideas are those that feed the soul with a healthful and true picture of reality.[2]

These truths are the bottom line to making dynamic and profound change in every dimension of your life. Identify your lies and replace them with new, healthy truths on a daily basis. Pray that God would reveal your misconceptions.

Once you identify the negative messages that are playing in your mind, take it one step further and reverse that message. What is the positive message you choose to believe instead? Write it down and repeat it each time you catch yourself having that negative thought. Don't stop this exercise until you fully believe the new message. Truly believing the new messages may take time, but it is worth the investment because it can powerfully change your life.

Be totally honest with yourself. What's the real reason for your personal challenges? Why do you lack motivation or commitment? What are the specific lies you believe? What new messages need to replace those lies?

Customize Your Self-Talk

If you want to change your thinking, take aggressive action and work on new messages. Whether you choose to "talk to yourself," make audio recordings, or simply meditate on truth, make sure you are using Scripture correctly within its appropriate context. Be sure other messages you have written are in harmony with the Word. Imagine how your life would change if you *really* believed those new truths. Do you suppose you would think and act differently if you repeated them several times a day for a full year? If the answer is yes, then do it! Read them, memorize them, repeat them until you feel as if your new, healthier lifestyle is now on automatic pilot. How long will that take? I don't know. I do know that you'll need to invest in your mind every day for the rest of your life. That is how you will grow and have victory in every dimension of your life.

Trigger Talk

Trigger talk is a useful technique that I teach women to use when they are trying to change their lifestyle habits. It is effective in any dimension of your life and will prompt you to repeat your customized self-talk several times each day. This is how it works: Identify an activity you engage in one or more times each day such as driving, looking at your watch, showering, or using the restroom. Use these events as "triggers" to remind you to repeat your new messages. For example, every time you turn the key to start your car, repeat your Scripture or new statement. At first, it will be difficult to remember to correlate a routine activity with your new habit of healthy thinking.

I call one of my most favorite triggers "potty talk." While most of us think of bad language as potty talk, I think of it as using time in the bathroom as a trigger to change my thinking. It makes sense. We all must use the bathroom several times each day. Most of us are rarely interrupted, and there's nothing else challenging our minds during this activity.

In our high-tech age, we can even use electronics to trigger us! I use my electronic day-timer by scheduling the alarm to go off three times a day when I want to memorize a new Scripture verse or form a new mental habit.

Just imagine how your focus in life would change if three times a day you were triggered to say something like this:

> "I am putting God first in my life. I am learning to love him with all my heart, soul, mind, and strength. I am loving my family, friends, and others as myself."

> "I choose to honor God with my body. I know that his Spirit lives within me, and I am remembering to ask him for help in dealing with temptations and changing my lifestyle."

One of the most helpful tools I have used in depositing life-changing truth into women's lives is a special self-talk tape that I created for weight loss many years ago. It incorporates more than forty Scripture passages and powerful truths to help my clients change their unhealthy thinking patterns related to their bodies and lifestyle habits. It is set to music and recorded in the first person as if the listener were speaking directly to

God. Hundreds of people have expressed that the tape is a powerful tool to help them transform their thinking.

Implementing Change

I recently got a call from a client who took my Scale Down . . . Live It Up program more than three years ago. She was calling to order new tapes because she had worn hers out completely! And she had lost more than one hundred pounds in the process. Today, Kathleen is helping facilitate our program in a very large church in San Diego and encouraging many women with the truth about how powerful change occurs when we change our minds.

The techniques used to change your thinking are simple. Yet doing so is difficult. We are creatures of habit and seem to easily forget what we have decided to do. Find creative ways to remind yourself to use your trigger until you get into the "trigger habit." Write your messages on the inside of your medicine cabinet, refrigerator door, or cupboard or put a Post-it note on your steering wheel. Do whatever it takes to remind yourself of your new activity.

Now, grab a pen and paper and complete the following exercise. Chances are that if you save it for later, it won't happen. Set yourself apart from the crowd and ensure victory by taking some action right now!

- Choose one or two triggers that you think will work best for you.
- Determine what reminders you will use to "trigger your triggers."
- Write down two to four statements or Scripture verses you believe will help you replace your unhealthy beliefs or thoughts.

- Memorize them.
- Make an effort and commitment to do this several times each day when you are triggered for a minimum of six months.

It's up to you to practice your new trigger talk until a change in your lifestyle becomes permanent. You will know it is permanent when two things occur.

First, your mind will automatically go there whenever you experience the trigger. Have you ever heard an old song and immediately been transported to a certain time or place in your life? It's as if you are watching a movie in your mind, the memories are so vivid. That is what will happen with your trigger. At some point, you won't even need to say your phrase or Scripture verse. Your trigger will take you there automatically.

Second, you'll know your trigger talk is effective when your feelings and behavior start to change. Since your mind believes what you tell it most often, your behavior and feelings will reflect that new belief. The challenge is to practice long enough for those changes to take place. It's up to you.

People tell me over and over that they truly believe that giving themselves new, healthier messages can really change how they think, feel, and behave. Yet, why then do so few actually follow through and initiate this behavior? I guess the simple answer is human nature. Sadly, we find it easier to stay in the comfort zone of unhealthy thinking and living than to take simple steps toward a victorious life. We often spend more time reading about change rather than actually making change.

You must want the benefit these changes will bring (like an energetic, lean body) in order to commit to anything different from your usual pattern of living. Make a commitment to spend at least ten minutes a day for the rest of your life investing in your mind. By doing this, you'll find yourself among a very small percentage of people who have defied the self-imposed limits of past experiences. With this in mind, I encourage you to step out of the "statistical average" and make a decision to take action.

HEALTH FLASH
TIPS FOR HOLY HOTTIES

Ginkgo Biloba

While many factors contribute to a healthy brain (especially the right balance of essential fatty acids as described in chapter 2), good circulation and nerve renewal are definitely near the top of the list. Ginkgo biloba helps promote both and much more. The leaves of the ginkgo, one of the oldest species of trees recorded, are the source for significant medicinals that have been used for centuries all over the globe.

Many researchers believe that ginkgo produces more antioxidant activity than many better known antioxidants such as vitamins C and E and beta-carotene. Several studies have shown that it exerts powerful antioxidant activity in the brain, eyes, and cardiovascular system. It is specifically helpful in treating:

1. Memory loss
2. Attention Deficit Disorder (related to concentration and memory, not hyperactivity)
3. Alzheimer's disease
4. Circulatory diseases
5. Depression

6. High blood pressure
7. Impotence
8. PMS
9. Radiation effects
10. Ringing in the ears
11. Stroke
12. Vision problems

Dr. Stengler recommends a standard dosage range from 120 to 360 milligrams a day. It can take up to eight weeks for a therapeutic benefit to be recognized.

Ginkgo protects blood vessels by reducing inflammation and can also be helpful in treating varicose veins. It is one of the best medicines in the world for improving circulation to the hands and feet. Remember when we were often cold b.h.f. (before hot flashes)?

Taking Action

1. What was the most important truth you gained from this chapter?
2. What changes, if any, do you desire to make related to that truth?
3. What specific thoughts or actions need to be implemented to make those changes?
4. What are your greatest stumbling blocks toward this change?
5. On a scale from one to ten (with ten being the highest) how important is this relative to other needs/changes in your life? Use this scale to help you create an overall action plan when you finish reading this book.

5

The Seasons of Our Lives

"For everything . . . turn, turn, turn . . . there is a season . . . turn, turn, turn . . . and a time for every purpose under heaven." Okay, I admit it. I heard this profound spiritual truth first on the radio in the '60s when the Byrds sang those words. In retrospect, they were probably the first Bible verses I could recite since I didn't grow up in a Christian home. Little did I know that the significance of these words would increase with each passing year. Read them now and embrace the memories of the seasons you have endured:

> For everything there is a season, and a time for every
> matter under heaven:
> A time to be born, and a time to die;
> a time to plant, and a time to pluck up what is
> planted;
> a time to kill, and a time to heal;
> a time to break down, and a time to build up;

a time to weep, and a time to laugh;
a time to mourn, and a time to dance;
a time to throw away stones, and a time to gather
 stones together;
a time to embrace, and a time to refrain from em-
 bracing;
a time to seek, and a time to lose;
a time to keep, and a time to throw away;
a time to tear, and a time to sew;
a time to keep silence, and a time to speak;
a time to love, and a time to hate;
a time for war, and a time for peace.

Ecclesiastes 3:1–8 NRSV

When I first heard those words, I reflected about college, career, love, marriage, and having babies. I didn't want to consider the flip side unless I absolutely had to. Daydreaming about the thrilling opportunities my future held was so much easier. However, in that same decade, we were entrenched in a controversial war in Vietnam, so, it was natural to relate to the words "a time for war, and a time for peace." We wondered how many more young people would die before the time for peace would come.

These were some of my thoughts during that era when another popular song called our time "The Age of Aquarius." I wanted to "let the sun shine in," but what I really needed in my "hippie" years was to let the "Son" shine in my life. That would come much later. Once "Turn, Turn, Turn" faded off the charts, I never gave the words another thought until years later.

Time flew by. My grandmother died when my first daughter was born. I experienced a challenging divorce and later met the man of my dreams. Rebellious children and successful careers filled the weeks and months. A year scarred with marital infidelity followed by reconciliation challenged my faith and strengthened my identity. I was learning by personal experience that there truly is a time for every matter under heaven. However, it wasn't until I hit my forties that I grasped how fleeting time really is. The days we spend on this earth are like a speck of sand in the ocean of eternity.

Time Is Fleeting

At 51 years, 8 months old as of this writing, I have already lived a whopping 18,870 days. That's 452,880 hours of eating, sleeping, blow-drying, laughing, crying, resting, striving, worshiping, and loving. Wow. I wonder how many more hours I have left.

I heard a story about a man who figured out a creative way to remind himself each week about the value of his life. After years of putting work and accomplishments ahead of family and God, he decided it was time to get his priorities in order. He realized that he had spent one Saturday too many on things that just didn't matter. One day he sat down and did a little arithmetic. Since on average most folks live to be about seventy-five, he figured that he had been allotted thirty-nine hundred Saturdays in his lifetime and he was going to live the rest to the max! He was fifty-five when he did this math, so he figured he had about a thousand of them left to enjoy.

The man went to a local toy store and bought every marble they had. In fact, he ended up visiting three toy stores to round up a thousand marbles. He took them home and put them in a clear plastic container. Every Saturday, he would take one out and throw it away. He found that by watching the marbles diminish, he could focus better on the more important aspects of his life. He said, "There is nothing like watching your time here on this earth running out to help get your priorities straight." When I heard the story, he had just taken the last marble out of the container. He figured if he could make it until the next Saturday, he was given a little "bonus" time. I've already used up 2,704 of my Saturdays. I think I'll start paying closer attention to my "marbles."

A Season of Contentment

Thirty-eight years have passed since I first heard "Turn, Turn, Turn." Today, as I reread the verses, I understand more profoundly the sweet and bitter realities of their meaning. I find it challenging some days to balance the harsh actualities of life with the eternal hope we have knowing the blessings God has stored up for us in heaven.

My personal prayer for this season is to have a heart of contentment and an attitude of surrender at all times. I wish I could say in all sincerity with the apostle Paul that "I have learned to be content in whatever circumstances I am" (Phil. 4:11). I can say I am "learning" present tense, but I cannot say I have "learned." Yet even as I write these words to you, I know that God is doing a good work in us. Together we are learning to embrace all he has given us as we pass the baton to those who will carry on. I want to say with Paul not only that I have *learned* to be content but also that "to live is Christ and to die is gain" (Phil. 1:21). That is the ultimate perspective I wish to achieve before I die.

Perhaps I am sounding a bit maudlin. Forgive me if that is true. But, these days I am compelled to ponder the more significant aspects of life. I'd rather do it now and make timely changes than regret on my deathbed that I had frittered away my most influential years.

How will you spend this very precious season of your life? Will you squander it away with busyness and nonsense?

Will you waste energy stressing about your less than perfect body or unfulfilled dreams? Try investing each moment you can in things that will matter for eternity. Live joyfully and passionately every day you have been given.

Many days, to start my day truly "on purpose," I spend a few minutes in prayer before I even get out of bed. That way, no matter what happens to my morning quiet time, I have begun by putting first things first. The verse that comes to my mind in those early hours is: "In the morning, O LORD, You will hear my voice; In the morning I will order my prayer to You and eagerly watch" (Ps. 5:3).

What do you pray as you begin each day? How do you purpose to live passionately for the Lord? Perhaps the following questions will give you new insights. They certainly have helped me find focus in this season of life:

1. If God revealed that you would die in one year, how would you live differently?
2. If time or money were no object, what changes would you make?
3. Why do *you* exist in this very time and place in this microcosm of eternity?
4. What is your purpose and how will you live it out?

If you've never taken the time to consider questions like these seriously, may I suggest that you do so very soon? Find a few hours (or better yet a full day) and ponder those possibilities. Why? Because the answers will very likely help you live a life of purpose. Hey, grab a pen and jot a few thoughts down beneath those questions. Go ahead; I've left you enough space.

There's a book for middle-aged men called *Halftime*. I think the guys are a bit delusional, gals. If they are over fifty, they are more likely in their last quarter of the game. No matter how many quarters, laps, seasons, or days we have left, it is essential that we live them to the fullest; not like some frenzied race to satisfy our wildest dreams but rather with a calm and purposeful commitment to let God use us to his glory every day we have left. *The Menopause Guide* is our handbook not just for "managing" menopause but for transforming our perspectives. Menopause is simply our daily reminder that every day is valuable.

Seize the Day!

"Seize the Day" is a beautiful song that challenges us to make the most of every moment God gives us. The chorus goes like this:

> Seize the day, seize whatever you can
> Cause life slips away just like hourglass sand[1]

I have a true hourglass. When I turn it over, in exactly one hour all the sand is drained to the bottom. Still. No motion. Time has run out.

Consider your last twenty-four hours. On a scale from one to ten, how would you rate the past day? Was it a downright miserable two? Maybe it was a delightful eight. Perhaps it was just an average day, whatever that means. Let's say average deserves a six. Or, if you had challenges at every turn, your day would receive a measly three on our scale. Go ahead— take a moment to give your day a grade. Your answer may tell you more than you might think. We'll address your score a little later.

In the movie *Dead Poets Society*, new teacher John Keating (played by Robin Williams) preaches to his English literature students at the exclusive Welton Academy. Standing on top of a classroom desk he exclaims, "Carpe diem, lads! Seize the day! Make your lives extraordinary!"

How does one "seize the day"? The true meaning of the Latin term *carpe diem* means to make the most of the moment. It also implies to some that you are to "do what you feel" without regard for the consequences. I would encourage you to seize each day, each moment *with* regard for the consequences. That is, make the most of celebrating life and honoring God with your attitude and actions.

Once we have satisfied our basic human needs for survival (food, clothing, and shelter), we have other emotional and spiritual needs that must be met in order to live life to the fullest. To deeply celebrate life despite our circumstances, we must focus on four essential needs:

1. Intimacy with God
2. Intimacy with others
3. A sense of significance
4. A sense of purpose

Seizing the day with an "abundance mentality" is recognizing that God is always in control. It is about knowing that his love for us is unconditional and perfect when we place our trust in him through faith in Christ. And, while we both celebrate and suffer in this temporal world, an attitude of abundance sees beyond today and looks to eternity with great hope that will never disappoint. Letting go of expectations and celebrating that which is often taken for granted is a big part of "seizing the day." Expectations dictate the way we think God's goodness should come to us—what kind of "box" life is supposed to come in. Here are a few suggestions that will help you develop realistic expectations and an accurate perspective on your life this very moment. Seize the day . . . every day, by:

- Reading the Word of God
- Spending time in prayer
- Dealing immediately with unresolved conflicts
- Addressing unresolved sin daily
- Developing meaningful connections with others
- Taking good care of your body
- Accomplishing at least one goal each day and celebrating it
- Giving something of yourself away (time, encouragement, laughter)

I AM A SUCCESS

I am a success today. My Father is the King!
He wraps his arms around me and gives me all good things.

Measured not in riches or those who know my name,
My success comes from loving the One who bore my shame.

I am a success today; though I sweat and toil and strain.
My energy and vision shall not all be in vain.

Traveling down life's road, the journey often breaks me.
Deep character he builds; his trials mold and shape me.

My vision burns with passion, a deep desire to share,
The Hope that is within me, with people everywhere.

True success is measured in living out HIS plan.
That is the lasting value of a woman or a man.

My dream is not impossible. I can live it every day,
Inspiring truth in lives I meet and touch along the way.

I AM a success today; the world need not know.
I need only my Savior's approval as I grow.

Life is rich, complex, and mysterious. Look up from your "to do" lists, frustrations, and challenges to rejoice about something in this very moment. Develop a mental focus that cultivates a heart of gratitude and thankfulness. Join with the psalmist in exclaiming, "This is the day which the LORD has made; let us rejoice and be glad in it" (Ps. 118:24). Notice, he didn't place any qualifications for rejoicing—if your friends are responsive to your needs; if your boss appreciates your hard work; if your husband gives you the attention you desire. When you have an attitude of joy, your influence to those around you is profound.

Now about that rating you gave your last day . . . if it wasn't an eight or higher, why not? Was it the day and all its circumstances or your perspective that needed changing? I have known people who have suffered with debilitating pain or heartbreak for long seasons and still they rejoiced and saw every day as a gift. Seize the day right now; take initiative and make each day a ten. It's up to you.

HEALTH FLASH

TIPS FOR HOLY HOTTIES

Healthy Hearts

The leading cause of death for women over fifty is from heart attacks. Also, because our hearts are smaller and our arteries more petite, a heart attack may cause more severe damage than what a man may experience. Don't let this hidden killer catch you by surprise. In the U.S., 200,000 women suffer heart attacks each year. The success rate with bypass surgery is reduced because our vessels are smaller and therefore more difficult to repair. That's one more reason for prevention being the key. Here are ten heart-healthy recommendations:

1. Eat seven to nine fruits and veggies daily.
2. Take in 25 grams or more of fiber each day.
3. Add essential fats (omega-3s) from nuts, olive oil, and coldwater fish to your diet or supplement.
4. Limit trans- and saturated fats.
5. Take a daily multivitamin supplement.
6. Get thirty minutes a day of aerobic activity.
7. Maintain a healthy size/weight.
8. Avoid tobacco completely (this is the single highest risk factor).
9. If you drink alcohol, limit it to no more than one drink per day on average.
10. Take control of undue stress in your life.

The Newest Testing Parameters

According to Dr. Mark Stengler, if you want an accurate assessment of your cardiovascular risk, ask your doctor to include the following tests on your next blood profile. They tell far more than standard cholesterol tests. Acting on any high risk factors now could save your life!

1. C-reactive protein
2. Homocystein
3. Fibrinogen
4. LPA
5. Fasting insulin

After having my cardiac blood profile, I was shocked to learn that on a scale from one to ten with ten being the worst, I had a risk factor of seven. That is because I have a high LPA genetic factor, which is a specific type of cholesterol that makes the arteries more prone to build up plaque. Despite my healthy lifestyle, this increases my cardiac risk significantly.

The good news is that I can decrease that risk by taking some key supplements such as CoQ10, large doses of vitamin E, and fish oil supplements. CoQ10 stands for Co-enzyme 10, which is a powerful antioxidant that improves cardiovascular health. Vitamin E is also an important antioxidant with the additional benefit of being a natural blood thinner, therefore helping prevent heart attack and stroke. The benefits of fish oil are profound, and I cover that in detail in the health flash section of chapter 2. I am so thankful that I became aware of this risk now, rather than relying on the false security of assuming I am a low risk because I eat well and exercise. Prevention is always the best medicine!

The Exercise Stress Test

Experts are realizing that the exercise stress test needs to be interpreted differently for women. Doctors need to measure two things: (1) how long a woman can continue to walk as the treadmill progressively speeds up, and (2) how quickly her heart rate returns to normal once she steps off. According to a twenty-year study led by Johns Hopkins University, women who score low on these two parameters are three and a half times more likely to die of heart disease than those who are in better cardiovascular condition. If you are over fifty or have any significant risks for heart disease, such as high blood pressure, high cholesterol, or obesity, ask your doctor to schedule this test. No procrastinating; call today!

Inflammation and Heart Disease

Time magazine's February 23, 2004, feature article was titled *"The Fires Within."*[2] It discussed in a nine-page article the latest advances in scientific research linking inflammation to a host of diseases including heart attacks, colon cancer, and Alzheimer's. In a 1997 study, people who were found to have the highest levels of C-reactive protein, a marker for chronic inflammation in the body, were three times as likely to suffer a heart attack in the next six years as those with the lowest levels.

There are many factors and theories about chronic inflammation that can lead to disease. I've noted one of the causes at the end of chapter 2 regarding the imbalance of the essential fatty acids omega-3 and omega-6. The solution to this one factor is simple: supplement. Another common cause of cardiovascular inflammation is poor gum health. Brushing and flossing well and seeing your dentist regularly are simple solutions.

Awareness

Though a lot has been written about women having atypical cardiac symptoms such as fatigue, nausea, or headache, chest pain is still the number one sign. However, many women dismiss their symptoms because they think heart attacks are primarily a risk for men. Thousands of women under forty die every year from sudden heart attacks. Don't assume you won't be one of those.

If you haven't had a comprehensive checkup in the last few years, make an appointment with your doctor after you finish this book. Start a list of questions and some of the tests you may want your doctor to order. Remember, as I've said elsewhere, you are the CEO of your health-care team. Make sure your doctor is on your team and that he knows you are well informed on the subject of your health. As a health professional, I am always amazed at how few questions people ask of their doctors. If yours doesn't have time to address your specific concerns, find one who will.

Taking Action

1. What was the most important truth you gained from this chapter?
2. What changes, if any, do you desire to make related to that truth?
3. What specific thoughts or actions need to be implemented to make those changes?
4. What are your greatest stumbling blocks toward this change?
5. On a scale from one to ten (with ten being the highest) how important is this relative to other needs/changes in your life? Use this scale to help you create an overall action plan when you finish reading this book.

6

You Go ... Go ... Go, Girl!

Remember when you used to say things like, "When the kids grow up, I'm going to spend more time on me"? For most of you that time has arrived, but you haven't slowed down one bit. The activities may be different (no more soccer mom car pools or making cupcakes for grade school birthday parties), but you're just as busy and perhaps more stressed out than you used to be, aren't you? If not, you can skip this chapter. No! Wait! I changed my mind. Read it and pass on the insights to a stressed-out friend over a nice relaxing cup of chamomile tea. That is if you can slow her down long enough to listen.

We need to stop ourselves now and then and ask this question: "Why am I doing what I'm doing?" With hormones raging and our body going through an almost reverse metamorphosis, we need a little "cocooning" time to nurture body, soul, and spirit. If we don't slow down and take care of ourselves in this season, we will not have the physical, mental, and emotional reserve to care for others.

Living without Margin

To foster inner peace, we need to create a little "margin" in our lives. In his book of the same title, Dr. Richard Swenson defines *margin* as the "white space" of life. Just imagine reading a book with one continuous run-on sentence:

> NowhitespacesNomarginsNopunctuationItwouldbesofrustratingandstressproducingThatiswhatlivingwithoutmarginisallaboutNocomfortzonesYoujustwanttoscreamletmeoffthiscrazymerrygoround!

Living without margin is being thirty minutes late to your doctor's appointment, because you were twenty minutes late meeting your business associate, because you ran out of gas two blocks from the gas station, because you were late getting home last night when you noticed your gas tank was close to empty and decided to wait until morning to fill up.

Life is like a rubber band. If you are stretched too often or too far, you eventually snap! So, are you stretched to your limit in any life areas? As Dr. Swenson writes:

> Living without margin is not having time to finish the book you're reading on stress. Margin is having time to read it twice. Living without margin is fatigue. Margin is energy. Living without margin is red ink. Margin is black ink. Living without margin is hurry. Margin is calm. Living without margin is anxiety. Margin is security.[1]

During the menopause madness phase of life (anywhere between thirty-five and fifty-five), we begin blaming most of our mental lapses and stressed-out moments on our hormone imbalance. In reality, much of our mental short-circuiting and many of our stresses have nothing to do with our age or hormones but rather with our lifestyle and perspectives. The brain is often compared to a computer. Most of us know how poorly our computer performs when we've overburdened it with too much info. If we have too many files or programs open at once, it bogs down, freezes up, or simply crashes. That is what we humans do as well . . . at any age!

I was reminded of how true this is when my seven-year-old grandson did something that reminded me of myself. After battling with a nasty sty in his left eye for weeks, we found out that washing the eyelid with baby soap would help resolve the infection more quickly. So, twice each day, Jesse would lather up his hands and rub the "no tears" bubbles on his eyelid and then wipe it dry. One morning, he was lagging getting ready for school and had to brush his teeth, wash his eyelid, and gel his hair all in less than five minutes. In his hurriedness and frustration, he began to wash his eye with Super Spiker Hair Gel. He caught himself millimeters from his eye and exclaimed, "How weird is that, Mom? I'm really getting silly; how did *that* happen?" Overload, my son, overload. And it can happen at any age when the margins of our life are reduced to the point that we are living on the edge of our mental, physical, and emotional capacity.

If you are an overachiever, the poem on the next page may help you "let go" and invest in memorable moments that touch and change lives for eternity. And by the way, if I'm sounding a tad bit condescending, it's only because I too spend more time *doing* than simply *being*.

More than thirty years ago, futurists predicted that due to technology we would have an abundance of spare time. Today,

YOUR DASH IN LIFE

I read of a man who stood to speak
At the funeral of a friend.
He referred to the dates on her tombstone
From the beginning . . . to the end.

He noted that first came her date of birth
And spoke that date with tears,
But he said what mattered most of all
Was the dash between those years.

For that dash represented all the time
That she spent alive on earth . . .
And now only those who loved her
Know what that dash was worth.

For it matters not, how much we own;
The cars . . . the house . . . the cash,
What matters is how we live and love
And how we spend our dash.

So think about this long and hard.
Are there things you'd like to change?
For you never know how much time is left,
That can still be rearranged.

If we could just slow down enough
To consider what's true and real,
And always try to understand
The way other people feel.

To be slower to anger,
Or show appreciation more,
And love the people in our lives
Like we've never loved before.

If we treat each other with respect,
And more often wear a smile . . .
Remembering that this special dash
Will only last a little while.

So, when your eulogy's being read
With your life's actions to rehash . . .
Would you be proud of the things they say
About how you spent your dash?

—Author Unknown

fax machines, once thought to be the cutting-edge way to get information relayed, are almost considered passé. Email and instant messaging are faster and more efficient. Cell phones are a common convenience. We get more done, faster than ever. But rather than choosing to use the time saved for relaxation and connection, we have simply increased our desires for greater productivity. From businesses to families . . . we are operating with "nanosecond" expectations. We are irritated by all the delays and distractions that occur on a daily basis. In fact, in a lifetime the average American will spend:

- six months sitting at traffic lights
- one year searching through desk clutter
- eight months opening junk mail
- two years calling people who don't answer
- five years waiting in line
- three years in meetings

Most of us would say, "What a waste of time!" And it is. Yet these time robbers are inevitable. Perhaps we need to change our thinking rather than learn new and more expedient ways to overcome these obstacles to our efficiency. There was a time in my corporate days when I exclaimed regularly, "There's just not enough hours in the day!" How arrogant of me to think I knew more about time management than God! God modeled for us the importance of rest, renewal, and balance. After six days of fashioning our universe, on the seventh he simply *rested*. He chose to demonstrate to us what he knew we needed to thrive in a fallen world living in frail and perishable bodies.

I love a quote I once heard that says, "What I do today is important because I am paying a day of my life for it.

What I accomplish must be worthwhile because the price is high." Sometimes the word *accomplish* is misunderstood. In God's economy, accomplishment is not about reaching all our worldly goals (not that those are bad things), but rather investing in worthwhile accomplishments that have eternal value. Most of us are so busy thinking about what we have to do that we don't think about what we want or *really* need to do.

Living with True Margin

So what *can* we do to restore some white space in our life that will ultimately lead to balance and deeper connection with our Creator and the people we love? In his book *Maximize the Moment*, T. D. Jakes says that overloaded people fail. Like an airplane, we can only hold so much luggage! When we expect too much or take on too much, we don't really do well at anything. He makes a simple yet profound statement that is a good recipe for the beginning of living with true margin: "To maximize your life . . . you must minimize your load!"[2]

That sounds good. But it's not easy. We have developed habits that support margin-less living. What's the answer? *Choose to change.* Minimize your load by practicing one of the first words you ever learned, "No!" Adding white space to your life will mean that on a daily (sometimes hourly) basis you will need to learn to choose the "best" from all the "good." Here are a few ways to decide if *anything* is worth your precious and limited time:

- Will it help me know and love God more?
- Will it help me know and love my spouse more?
- Will it help me know and love my children more?

• Will it help me grow in loving others more?

Sometimes it is important to "get back to basics" and implement some simple principles of what I call "on-purpose" living. Here are a few reminders (you already know these truths) that will help you restore both time and emotional margin in your life.

Restoring the Time Margin

1. Expect the unexpected. Increase your time window in all your plans to decrease the rush.
2. Learn to say no (and mean it)!
3. Prune your activities to essentials whenever you can.
4. Release yourself from our fast mentality (and release others also).
5. Look up and out—see the vision of the bigger picture.
6. Get less done, but do the right things!
7. Create your own buffer zones—schedule your free time for both daily and weekly renewal.

Restoring Emotional Margin

1. Establish meaningful friendships; you need close friends to share your highest and lowest moments.
2. Express yourself honestly—laugh and cry.
3. Maintain healthy boundaries with the people in your life.
4. Develop an attitude of gratitude. Just think how happy you would be if you lost everything you now have and then suddenly got it back!
5. Ask yourself this question: "What is the worst thing that could happen if . . ."

I received this "memo from God" some time ago via email. It was on a day that I needed some reminders of how to keep life in perspective as I scurried about impatiently, becoming irritated at every inconvenient glitch in my personal agenda. Perhaps when you are experiencing the "too much to do, too little time" syndrome, this memo will help you make the transition from "go, go, go" to "being still" and knowing he is God.

—Memo from God

I am God. Today I will be handling all of your problems. Please remember that I do not need your help.

If life happens to deliver a situation to you that you cannot handle or is out of your control, do not attempt to resolve it. Kindly put it in an imaginary box labeled "SFGTD" (something for God to do). It will be addressed in my time, NOT yours. Once the matter is placed into the box, do not hold on to it.

Here are some other directions for today:

1. If you find yourself stuck in traffic, don't despair. There are people in the world for whom driving is an unheard privilege.

2. Should you have a bad day at work, think of the man or woman who has been out of work for a long time.

3. Should you despair over a relationship that has ended, think of the person who has never known what it's like to love and be loved in return.

4. Should you grieve the passing of another weekend, think of the woman in dire straits, working twelve hours a day, seven days a week to feed her children.

5. Should your car break down, leaving you miles away from assistance, think of the paraplegic who would love the opportunity to take that walk.

6. Should you notice a new gray hair in the mirror, think of the cancer patient in chemo who wishes she had hair to examine.

7. Should you find yourself the victim of other people's bitterness, ignorance, rudeness, or insecurities, remember things could be worse. You could be them.

8. I love you and care about every detail of your life. If you care more about others, you'll see your trials in perspective.

9. Give those difficulties then to me. Put them in the box and move on!

The Power of Choice

In mentoring men about balancing life and priorities, Edmond Louis Cole once said, "Everything is under the power of choice, but once a choice is made, we become a servant to that choice." It's not just the men who need help in this area. We need to take a hard look at why and where we spend our time. If we cannot honestly say that our busyness is tied to things that make a difference, then we need to question why we are doing what we're doing.

Sometimes it takes a lot of work and "undoing" to make up for a poor or misguided choice. For example, we cannot simply decide to quit our jobs because we are tired of the rat race of the corporate world, if our income is responsible for a certain percentage of the bills. We need to take reasonable steps toward change at the same time taking responsibility for less than ideal choices. That is played out over and over in America as frustrated families pay thousands of dollars to their credit card companies each year.

I've made some poor choices over the years that I've regretted deeply. In 1997, my business partner, Terri, and I decided we needed a nice office with a classroom to allow us to do our seminars "in house." We hired a consultant, prayed about the decision, and made a foolish assumption that just because "the door opened" and the lease was approved, God had blessed our decision. But it ended up being foolish and costly. When we realized our plans and priorities were off track, we wanted to make some immediate changes. But it just wasn't that simple.

We need to be very careful of the commitments we make, as they are not always easily undone. In fact, it took Terri and me more than three years to find a lasting solution to the reality of our *five*-year lease. Fortunately, we were able to sublease our space and cut our losses after we surrendered to the fact that our hanging in there "on faith" was not God's plan for a healthy business but rather our idealistic thinking.

Change is difficult. If it weren't, we'd all be perfect. You probably *know* the right choices you need to make. But, if you're not sure, seek wise counsel, study God's Word, and pray for the wisdom to know *and* choose the best from all the good. Remember, too many "good" things add up to a chaotic and marginless life. Don't run through life so fast that you forget not only where you've been but also where you are going.

Psalm 46:10 says, "Be still, and know that I am God" (NIV). But how many of us live it? What does it really mean to "be still"? It's interesting to note that the NASB says this: "Cease striving and know that I am God." The Hebrew word that "be still" and "cease striving" are translated from, *raphah*, means to abate, cease, be feeble, idle, leave, let alone, slack, be still or weak.

So what is God telling us? We need to slow down, be quiet, and realize our complete weakness without him. By acknowledging our feebleness, we can see his immensity, perfection, and sovereignty more clearly. It is in this realization that we begin to comprehend the futility of our striving and busyness. It is in this comprehension of the eternal perspective that we can let go of the anxiety and frustrations of daily living and find peace and joy in the midst of life's storms.

Got stress? Get rest! Rest for your body, soul, and spirit. The best place to start is to simply cease striving, present your requests and prayers with a heart of thanksgiving, and dwell on that which is pleasing in God's sight. Then his peace will overcome the stresses of your day.

HEALTH FLASH
TIPS FOR HOLY HOTTIES

R & R for Your Body and Soul

God designed us with a mind that needs down time, a soul that needs refreshment, and a body that needs sleep within every twenty-four-hour cycle. According to experts, sleep is when our body's best cellular regeneration occurs. Why do we fight God's design and think it is noble to work like crazy and run at a frantic pace? It's been said that stress kills. While a certain amount of stress is healthy and moves us forward, too much does "kill" us both physiologically and psychologically. Our busy lifestyles are not normal even though we may not know anything different. We must begin to recognize the value of true rest. I love what Jesus said to the disciples when they had been overwhelmed by people coming and going without even having time to eat. He told them, "Come away by yourselves to a secluded place and rest a while" (Mark 6:31).

A year ago, my husband and I partnered up with our pastor and my parents and bought a little log cabin in the mountains near Big Bear Lake, California. That is where I often go to write, slow down, or simply enjoy nature by myself or with family and friends.

Nature has an astonishing way of slowing us down and calming our souls. But getting away physically is not always practical. We need to learn how to take mini-retreats for mind and body right in the middle of our daily lives.

1. Take a warm bath by candlelight with soft praise music playing.
2. At the first sign of anxiety or stress, take a few slow, deep breaths in through your nose and out through your

mouth and remind yourself that most things are simply not worth the importance we assign them.

3. Turn down the lights in your office, put a warm towel over your shoulders to relax the muscles, prop up your feet, and close your eyes for five luxurious minutes.

4. Exercise daily for increased energy, decreased stress, and maximum wellness.

5. Play soothing music in your car and focus on relaxing all your muscles from head to toe while you're driving in traffic. Tell yourself that you can't make the traffic move any faster, so you may as well slow down internally and go with the flow.

6. Lie on the floor and stretch your body as long as you can, tensing up every muscle. Then slowly, starting at your toes, release all the tension. Take a few slow, deep breaths and blow off the stresses of the day.

7. Choose peace. Set your mind on things above, and you will be astonished at how the focus of your mind and the power of God can bring a peace that truly passes all understanding. God rested on the seventh day as an example to us.

Restoring physical margin requires that we take personal responsibility for our health and body. It will blow your mind when you realize how much better you can feel when you make small changes in your habits and responses to stress.

You may be thinking, *Danna, you don't know how stressful things are in my life right now. It's impossible not to worry.* I don't doubt that many reading these pages have burdensome pressures to address. When I struggle with things that are out of my control, I go to this verse and realize that Paul gave no caveats regarding the right to stress out. He says: "Be anxious for nothing, but in everything by prayer and supplication with thanksgiving let your requests be made known to God. And the peace of God, which surpasses all comprehension, will guard your hearts and your minds in Christ Jesus" (Phil. 4:6–7).

There is a powerful formula for dealing with stress and worry in this passage. Paul doesn't simply tell us not to be anxious, he gives us something productive to do instead: pray with a thankful heart. While your mind races and you are trying to relax or get to sleep, cry out to your God who hears every word. Tell him your pain, state your requests, and thank him that he knows even better than you what you really need. Trust him to supply that need according to his perfect timing and purpose. The promise is not that he will answer exactly as you ask; it is that his peace will guard your heart and mind. That means, when we truly give him all our "stuff," he takes it on and we can relax in a true peace knowing that our loving heavenly Father has it covered. Now relax, girlfriend. It's good for your soul.

Taking Action

1. What was the most important truth you gained from this chapter?
2. What changes, if any, do you desire to make related to that truth?
3. What specific thoughts or actions need to be implemented to make those changes?
4. What are your greatest stumbling blocks toward this change?
5. On a scale from one to ten (with ten being the highest) how important is this relative to other needs/changes in your life? Use this scale to help you create an overall action plan when you finish reading this book.

7

Get a Lifestyle—Eating and Living for Maximum Energy in the *Real* World

Do you have all the energy you want to live life to the fullest? Is your body lean and well toned? Are you free of chronic aches, pain, or disease? If the answer is yes, congratulations! You are the exception, and you can skip the next three chapters. But most women struggle with any number of lifestyle issues such as eating nutritiously, exercising regularly, or minimizing stress in their lives. Most are not living with maximum health and vitality.

A strong foundation in the basics is essential. Before trying every menopause herb and supplement on the market, make sure your lifestyle is on the right track. Too many people jump to pills to take away symptoms without considering that a vitally healthy (albeit aging) body handles natural changes like menopause most effectively. If you could visit with your great-grandmother, you might find out that her menopausal symptoms were much less severe than yours. Why? Most likely her diet was more nutritious, her activity level was higher, and her exposure to pollutants was limited. Our challenge is to try our best to recapture a lifestyle more like Great-Grandma's. We also need to learn how to detoxify our bodies and environments as best we can.

Several years ago, *Don't Sweat the Small Stuff*, a small book with a big impact, gave great advice about letting go of things that really don't matter—especially the things that stress us out. But in the physical dimension it *is* the small stuff that counts; the little things we do every day really matter. My lifestyle motto is this: small steps taken consistently add up in a big way over time!

If you read my first book, *Scale Down*, you know about my battle of the body, which began in my early teens. For decades everything I pursued in the physical dimension was for the sole purpose of gaining or maintaining a leaner body. I dieted, exercised, and popped pills based on what impact those might have on my outward appearance. Sadly, most of us are motivated first by our looks and second by our health. Not until we start feeling the impact of our poor choices do we truly get motivated to do the right things for the right reasons.

Let me encourage you to evaluate your lifestyle and make your body a priority . . . for health's sake. Romans 12:1 says, "Offer your bodies as living sacrifices, holy and pleasing to God—this is your spiritual act of worship" (NIV). My body can be a pleasing sacrifice? Why does Paul say this? We know that when we come to Christ, the Holy Spirit takes residence in our bodies and we become his temple (see 1 Cor. 3:16). While many references about our bodies are related to sexual purity, we are nevertheless his temple in all aspects of our physical existence. We have been "bought with a price." This "vehicle" we're driving through life is on loan. I believe we honor God when we treat it with the utmost respect. That includes our daily lifestyle choices.

Throughout this book, I give health tips specific to menopause. From dealing with hot flashes and mood swings to low libido and depression, there are many natural ways to minimize the manifestations of menopause. But a healthy lifestyle is the foundation needed for these natural remedies to truly work to their maximum potential.

With that in mind, I am ready to give you a crash course in the basics. If you simply apply the principles you learn in these next few pages *consistently*, you will be surprised at how much better you will look and feel.

When I teach nutrition, I always remind people that it is a "soft science." What I mean is that there are many theories and ideas out there at any given time. Experts seem to be constantly contradicting each other. If it were that complicated to eat healthfully, God would have created us with a "user's manual." While there are some teachings in the Bible that are helpful, you don't find many "Thou shalt not eat sugar" type of statements. And as New Testament believers we can celebrate with Paul the law of liberty, which states: "All things are lawful for me, but not all things are profitable. All things are lawful for me, but I will not be mastered by anything" (1 Cor. 6:12).

This verse is a wonderful prescription for living in all dimensions of our lives. While God has given us the blessing of our senses to see, feel, hear, taste, and smell—we don't need to overindulge those "senselessly." There is always a price to pay when we allow ourselves to become "mastered" by our flesh. When we enjoy all God has given us to live healthfully in moderation, our bodies respond wonderfully.

When I try to figure out the best way to eat and live, I try to imagine how people lived hundreds or even thousands of years ago. They didn't need a nutritionist or doctor to tell them how to live. They ate the foods God made available. By necessity they lived very active lifestyles and slept when natural light was no longer available. The answers are simple. We know them. We just choose not to live them out.

In my book *Scale Down: A Realistic Guide to Balancing Body, Soul, and Spirit*, I went into great detail about how to eat for maximum health and energy in the real world. To help women grasp the simplicity of eating healthfully, I came up with a simple "formula" called the NutriMax Six. I have reviewed it in part in this chapter. If your health, energy, or weight are challenges in your life, I encourage you to dig into these issues in depth in *Scale Down*. For the rest of you, simply start notching up your nutritional habits a bit in each area over the next year, and you might actually think you've turned back your age clock a few years . . . maybe even a full decade; because it's true what they say; you really are what you eat!

The NutriMax Six

It is my experience that most women take an all-or-nothing approach to nutrition and dieting. That is, they are either on a "health binge" or off. If you get one thing out of this chapter, I hope it is that small improvements made daily will truly add up. It's more beneficial to improve your nutrition by 10 or 20 percent for the rest of your life than it is to eat perfectly for a month or two and then fall back into your old habits. In chapter 10 you will have an opportunity to evaluate your nutritional habits and design a plan to begin a new lifestyle. Determine which two or three things are the most important or what you can even handle right now. Start there and add more changes as you are ready.

NutriMax #1: Water

These days, everyone *knows* that they need lots of good quality water on a daily basis. Yet few consistently get all they need. In fact, my friend and world-renowned author of *Prescription for Nutritional Healing*, Dr. James Balch, says that most people are running around with subclinical dehydration.

Your body doesn't sweat soda or iced tea; it sweats water and electrolytes. It needs water to perform all of its bodily functions. When you don't drink enough, your body resorts to handling only the most essential functions first . . . and that is not metabolizing excess fat! Try to drink at least four to eight ounces of water for every hour you are awake. If you wait to drink it until you're thirsty, you're already a quart low (four cups). Only water can be drawn directly into your cells from the gut without going through a "filtering process." All other beverages must first be "cleaned up" before entering your bloodstream.

When you get a headache, feel low energy, or even just feel hungry, try a big glass of pure water and see what happens. It is often exactly what the doctor ordered. Limit your intake of water from disposable plastic bottles. The material they are made from is very unstable. Never refill them, because by doing so you increase the intake of microscopic plastic particles even more. What you can't see *can* hurt you. If you want to look younger, have more energy, and live longer, drink pure, fresh water all day long!

NutriMax #2: Plant Foods

Multitudes of studies show increasing evidence that diets high in plant foods (fruits, vegetables, legumes, whole grains, and nuts) will have the most profound long-term effect on your health and vitality. Supplements cannot completely fill in the gaps left from not eating enough live, whole foods. The fiber in plant foods has an incredible balancing effect on blood sugar, not to mention the fabulous benefits to your entire digestive system. And don't forget that your breads and cereals should have enough whole grains to actually be considered "food." Most refined, packaged foods enter the body and are pretty much turned to sugar and paste within minutes of ingestion. Wonder why you feel so sluggish?

Fiber-rich fruits, vegetables, whole grains, beans, legumes, seeds, and nuts are packed with phytochemicals, antioxidants, and fiber. All three help fight cancer, provide anti-aging protection, and more. In fact, fiber in every meal will slow the release of the carbohydrates into your bloodstream and help you maintain a high energy level all day long. It will also minimize the overproduction of insulin triggered by too much refined carbohydrates, which leads to increased fat storage as your body strives to keep blood sugar levels in check.

Mom was right to encourage you to eat more of these foods. Now that you're not under her watchful eye, how are you doing on your own? And if you are a mom, how are your kids doing? The old recommendation to have seven to nine fruit and vegetable servings daily is still great advice.

With the craze toward protein diets, many people avoid "high glycemic" fruits and vegetables such as bananas, apples, potatoes, and corn. Think about all the incredible foods God created that are not allowed on the Atkins or other high-protein diets. It's as if we are saying, "Hey, God, why didn't you consult Dr. Atkins *before* you made all those foods? Didn't you know how bad they are for us?" The reality is this: if we ate as we were designed to with balance and moderation, we wouldn't be fat. By taking a whole group of foods out of our diets, we miss many key nutrients. That, however, does not diminish the reality that we simply eat too much food, especially processed products in bags, boxes, and cans.

NutriMax #3: Protein

Want high energy? Make sure you get an excellent source of protein at both breakfast and lunch. Like fiber, protein is essential for blood sugar control and can make a huge impact in your sweet cravings as well. Over the years, I have had clients share excitedly again and again how much this one dietary guideline has helped them lose weight and gain control over fatigue.

Protein is essential for tissue repair, maintenance, and growth of muscles, blood, hormones, enzymes, and antibodies. The reason that protein stabilizes your blood sugar and makes you feel satiated longer is because it digests very slowly. One of the reasons protein diets are so popular is that people have learned that it is harder to turn excess protein calories into fat. The conversion from protein to fat "burns up" about 40 percent of the excess calories in the process. Sounds like a good reason to eat lots and lots of protein, right? Wrong! Too much protein can overtax your body, particularly wreaking havoc on your kidneys. In addition, too much red meat has been linked in some studies to increased risk of osteoporosis. And an excess in any key nutritional area means you have to decrease in another key area, leaving your body with a significant nutritional gap.

To determine your average need for protein, divide your weight in half. If you weigh 140 pounds, you need at least 70 grams of protein each day. People on low-carbohydrate, high-protein diets are getting 200 to 400 or more grams each day. This is very hard on the body as it takes a lot more enzymes and other factors to digest protein than it does carbohydrate or fat.

Try to get as much protein as you can from plant sources such as beans, legumes, and nuts. In addition to fiber, phytochemicals, and antioxidants, these nutrient-dense foods are packed with protein. Ideally, take in at least 15 to 20 grams of protein at both breakfast and lunch. Also find creative ways to add a little protein to your snacks with nuts, peanut butter on whole-grain crackers, and so on.

Some scientists believe that Asian menopausal women experience few negative symptoms and enjoy better bone health because of their high soy intake. Japanese women, for example, consume approximately 100 to 200 milligrams a day—far more than their American counterparts—and suffer far fewer menopausal symptoms. In those cultures there is no word for hot flashes or PMS because the women there don't experience them. That is unless they become Americanized and start eating like we do.

Soy's phytoestrogens are thought to give the plant its hormone-balancing properties. One twelve-week study of postmenopausal women found that consuming 60 grams of soy protein daily (containing 76 milligrams of isoflavones) resulted in a 45 percent reduction in daily hot flashes. Some women noticed their hot flashes diminishing within five days of adding soy to their diets. Eating soy can also help relieve vaginal dryness, improve bone density, and balance cholesterol levels.

The studies that have validated soy's benefits have been conducted on people who consume actual soy foods such as miso, tofu, tempeh, and others. Until isolated soy supplements are studied more in depth, we cannot be sure of their comparable effectiveness. One of the easiest ways to add soy to your diet daily is to use soy milk in a morning protein shake, on your cereal, or in your coffee. If you experience gas and bloating when eating soy, try supplemental enzymes to help prevent this problem.

NutriMax #4: Fats

Fats have long been getting a bad rap, but the truth is that some are essential to your health. The key is to eat the right kind of fat, because, as with carbohydrates, not all fats are created equal.

In the past year, I have come to realize that perhaps one of the single biggest nutritional gaps in the American diet is the lack of omega-3 fatty acids as I discussed in chapter 2. This essential fat impacts brain function and cardiac health dramatically and has been linked to positive protection from Alzheimer's disease. And, as I mentioned before, it is terrific for your skin . . . a wonderful benefit for menopausal women!

Choosing the right fats and understanding their benefits and drawbacks will help you dramatically in your weight management efforts. Keeping the proper amount of healthy fat in your diet will leave you feeling satiated longer than a nonfat meal.

Lots of people simply eat too much fat. For now, try to reduce the saturated (animal and dairy) fats in your diet as much as possible. The total fat in your diet should range between 15 and 30 percent. Stay on the lower end until you reach your ideal body fat goal. Olive oil is always a good choice for cooking and salads. As stated before, you can add omega-3 fats by eating coldwater fish like salmon; walnuts and flaxseed are also very high in omega-3 fat. Most people need to supplement to meet the recommended daily allowance because they don't get enough in their food.

In the last decade, the food industry has shifted from its use of saturated fats, lard, and oils to the "healthier" omega-6 vegetable oils. While omega-6 fats are considered essential, the problem today is that we are getting 15 to 20 times more than we need. As I mentioned before, this disparity between our omega-3 and 6 fats is creating a major problem in our bodies leading to significant inflammation in our joints, cardiovascular systems, and even brain tissue. Beware that most of the snacks and products you eat out of bags and boxes are drenched in vegetable oil. One way to improve the balance is to use olive oil, which is an omega-9 fat, in as much of your cooking as possible.

NutriMax #5: Vitamins

God provides all the nutrients we need in natural foods. The problem is that we don't eat the amount and variety of whole foods necessary to meet all of our nutritional needs. We also have corrupted our natural food sources with depleted soil, polluted water, and chemical agents such as pesticides.

Vitamins and minerals are essential nutrients that occur naturally in foods yet provide no calories. Antioxidants are a specific group of nutrients that together form an army that captures the metabolic waste products called free radicals and transports them out of your body before they can damage your cells. All these "micronutrients" act like spark plugs, working to help your body perform its various functions effectively. They also help you utilize your food as fuel more effectively and prevent nutritional deficiencies.

Today, it's important to take vitamins and minerals as an insurance policy in your diet. However, they do not take the place of healthy eating. Just as new spark plugs won't make your car run better if you forget to put gasoline in your car, vitamins without good food are of little value. If you're not already taking vitamins, start with a good multivitamin mineral complex and an antioxidant formula. Then, if you have a specific need, supplement based on the recommendations of your health-care professional. A word of wisdom: don't spend a fortune on micromanaging your nutrition before you get the

basics down. Make the the NutriMax Six a consistent habit
. . . *then* start fine-tuning.

NutriMax #6: Vitamins Z and X

Okay, I know . . . I know . . . the next two "nutrients" aren't
nutrients at all. But, they are essential to ensuring your body
is a high-energy machine. If you eat perfectly every day and
miss these two vital components, you simply cannot have the
health and vitality you desire.

Vitamin Z—better known as sleep—is an often-neglected
"nutrient" that plays a much more important role in our
health than we previously realized. Sleep is the time when
you get both physical and psychological rest. During deep
sleep, your body accomplishes its most important cellular
renewal. Even modest amounts of sleep deprivation can
diminish your immune system and ability to cope with the
daily challenges of life. If you want to look younger, feel
better, and live longer . . . get enough sleep! How much is
enough? Experts suggest that most people need close to eight
hours of sleep every night. I have found that chronic fatigue
is one of the biggest factors impacting an out-of-control
appetite. I think your body is basically saying, "If you're
not going to give me enough quality rest to reenergize,
I'm just going to beg for sugar and calories all day long to
make up for it!" My suggestion: make sleep a priority. Try
it for a full month and see for yourself the impact it makes
in your lifestyle.

Vitamin X—better known as exercise—is essential for
maintaining high energy, low body fat, and overall health and
vitality. I will cover this topic fully in chapter 8. For now, let
me leave you with an important thought that will motivate you
to move more. Exercise is an incredible energizer. The more
you move, the better you feel. Feeling good motivates you to

stay active, and activity tends to distract you from sedentary habits that include eating. Get in a positive cycle and get a good dose of vitamin X every day!

Top Ten Supplements

With so many supplements on the market, we could easily spend several hundred dollars *each month* and still not know if we are taking the right ones. I have designed the following top ten list with Dr. Mark Stengler. It includes vitamins, herbs, and specialty whole food supplements. Obviously, this list may leave out some things that may be helpful to specific individual health concerns, but I do think it is a good starting place for the average person. While many people don't want to buy or ingest ten different products, Dr. Stengler definitely recommends including the first three in every family's supplement regime. In this list, I have briefly detailed the key benefits of each supplement.

1. High-Potency Vitamin-Mineral Complex

Busy lifestyles, poor eating habits, and the diminished quality of our food make supplementation a necessity in this day and age. Of course, supplementation is always secondary to eating as nutritiously as possible. A quality vitamin-mineral complex should be taken in at least two doses for maximum absorption. Capsule and liquid formulas ensure your supplement is absorbed. As a rule of thumb, don't buy the cheapest or most expensive products on the market. With the first, you are most likely giving up quality, and for the latter, you may be paying a premium for marketing methods or "hype." Find a good midrange price from a reputable company that has been offering products for some time.

2. Super Green Foods

Super green foods such as wheat grass, barley grass, alfalfa, spiralina, chlorella, and kelp are excellent sources of real foods that enhance our health in multiple ways including detoxification, increased immune function, blood sugar stabilization, and increased energy. Despite their plant base, super green foods are an excellent source of protein that is highly bio-available. They also are great natural and readily absorbable sources of calcium. (Believe it or not, dairy products are not the best source.)

3. Essential Fatty Acids

Want to have a sharp mind and great skin? The essential fatty acids, omegas 3, 6, and 9, are the nutrients you need on a daily basis. Limited food sources for these important nutrients include cold-water fish such as salmon, walnuts, pecans, almonds, flaxseed, and a few green leafy vegetables such as kale and bok choy. Since it is unrealistic for most people to get adequate amounts in their diets, supplementation is essential. It is also important to note that most of us are getting too much omega-6 because of the ingestion of so many vegetable oils. Olive oil is high in omega-9 and should be used as much as possible to counteract this imbalance, which increases the inflammatory response throughout the body. See chapter 2 for more detailed information on this subject.

4. Vitamin C

While most animals can manufacture their own vitamin C, humans need to get it in their diets. A potent antioxidant with great immunity-boosting effects, it also has some of its own unique characteristics. For example, vitamin C is required for the production of collagen. It strengthens capillaries and may be helpful for those who bruise easily. It also is very helpful in dealing with arthritis because of its anti-inflammatory properties. As a cancer-fighting agent, vitamin C protects the genetic material in cells (DNA) from damage. The average person can take at least 2,000 milligrams per day in divided doses.

5. Garlic

Garlic is one of the most researched herbs in the world and has extraordinary attributes both as a food and a supplement. Its main medicinal benefits include cardiovascular protection, improved cholesterol levels, lowered blood pressure, diminished blood-clotting, improved circulation, and protection against cancer and infectious diseases.

6. Calcium/Magnesium

Calcium is required by every cell of your body for a variety of actions including muscle contraction, healthy nerves, cell division, and the release of neurotransmitters that scoot between nerve cells, not to mention healthy bones and teeth. Only 10 percent of adults get enough calcium each day; most children are falling short as well. Caffeine, alcohol, and sugar all promote urinary excretion of calcium. Hormone imbalances and poor digestive function can also contribute to calcium deficiency. From eight years old to eighty, most people need at least 1,000 milligrams a day of good quality calcium, which is best absorbed in 500-milligram doses with 250 milligrams of magnesium. You can find some quality supplements that are a combination of calcium and magnesium in the proper ratio.

7. Vitamin E

Vitamin E is found in the fats of most vegetables and grains. Unfortunately, processing foods destroys this vital nutrient that provides antioxidant properties as well as important support to the nervous system, muscle function, and overall healing. People with diseases such as diabetes, Parkinson's disease, fibrocystic breast syndrome, and multiple sclerosis should have extra vitamin E supplementation. The average adult should take 400 IU daily. The best source to look for is alpha-tocopherol.

8. Ginkgo Biloba

This mighty little plant is something Dr. Stengler prescribes on a daily basis to treat a wide range of conditions— from memory impairment and dizziness to headaches and depression. It has an extraordinary ability to increase circulation to the brain and extremities. Its natural blood-thinning effects are important to the prevention of strokes and heart attacks. He suggests 60 milligrams two to four times per day. Individuals with early-stage Alzheimer's disease should take 240 to 360 milligrams daily.

9. Green Tea

With about half the amount of caffeine as coffee, green tea provides a reasonable energy boost without the sharp "ups and downs" of coffee and its calcium-robbing effects. It is a great antioxidant and anti-cancer agent that also helps the liver with detoxification, which is essential for balancing hormones and cleansing the body of many forms of toxins. Preliminary research shows that green tea can help stabilize blood sugar and thus indirectly promote weight loss by preventing insulin spikes. Green tea extract is available in liquid and capsule forms.

10. Milk Thistle

Most people in America have significant toxins in their bodies, and their livers are overburdened. Our bodies are not equipped to deal with the staggering amount of chemicals that bombard us on a daily basis. Milk thistle is a potent herb that works specifically in the protection and revitalization of the liver. It also stimulates good digestion of fats as well as improves elimination. Dr. Stengler recommends one 250-milligram capsule three times a day.

HEALTH FLASH

TIPS FOR HOLY HOTTIES

Seven Nutritional Steps You Can Take Right Now

1. Don't try to micromanage your nutrition. Get the basics down first.
2. Eat as well as you can every day by practicing the NutriMax Six.
3. Keep supplementation simple. More is not always better.
4. Listen to your body—it will tell you how you are doing.
5. Seek professional help if you aren't at peak health.
6. Keep a reasonable and healthy perspective.
7. Remember, every small improvement counts!

God put us in these corporeal "tents" for the years we spend on earth. The quality of our life will be directly associated with our level of health. It is hard to live life to the fullest when we don't feel full of energy and vitality.

Genetics and circumstances are out of our control. Yet more than 70 percent of our health will depend upon our lifestyle. Taking good care of ourselves by practicing good nutrition will have a huge impact on how well we function for the next few decades.

8

Exercise—Use It or Lose It!

Women ask me all the time, "How much do I really need to exercise? If I don't have a weight problem, how important is it?" Here is the bottom line: God designed us for movement . . . every day . . . for a lifetime. If you don't purposely bend, stretch, lift, pull, walk, skip, row, bike, and climb in your normal daily activities, then you better start simulating those motions in what is now termed "exercise."

We think that our sedentary lifestyles are normal and that getting a fifteen-minute aerobic workout a few times a week is sufficient. While it is certainly better than nothing, true health and vitality comes from consistently telling your bones, muscles, and joints, "I need you!" That is, use them or they will degenerate and you will age prematurely.

Now, that being said, you don't need to overdo it either. In fact, too much of a good thing ages you prematurely as well. When we exercise like fanatics, our bodies have to work overtime processing all the free radicals that are expended as we consume more oxygen for all the activity. As I have and will say again and again, balance, moderation, and consistency are the key in *every* lifestyle area.

The Big Picture

Have you ever noticed that once you get moderately fit and over the initial aches, pains, and out-of-shape blues, exercise becomes invigorating? It becomes a positive energy merry-go-round. The more you move, the better you feel. Feeling good motivates you to stay active, and activity tends to distract you from sedentary habits that include eating. Many people report feeling less stress, irritation, depression, and anxiety following regular exercise. There are also the extra benefits of improved self-esteem, mood, and an enhanced ability to concentrate; these result in part from endorphins, chemicals in the body that give you a "high" feeling after exercise. Endorphins also help relieve body aches and pains. In some studies, women who exercised regularly were less prone to hot flashes. More important, to prevent osteoporosis, you need to stimulate bone growth through a weight-bearing activity such as walking.

Almost every physical problem from insomnia to fibromyalgia or heart disease to diabetes is positively influenced by an active lifestyle. Our bodies were designed for daily movement. This reality becomes more essential as we age. While I've been active for decades, I am finding that I lose my muscle tone faster than ever. If I don't move purposely almost every day to keep fit, I can almost see myself going backward. And, despite the fact that I ski fast and furious like a twenty-year-old, it's a fifty-two-year-old achy body that needs an hour in the hot tub after a day on the slopes.

Fit Bodies

In the journey to fine-tune your fitness to your desired level, you can apply some basic principles I will outline below that will help you toward your goal. Think of your need for exercise as just as essential as your need for food and water. Lifestyle fitness is about getting in tune with your body and making some decisions about what you want and need it to do for you. Decide to make exercise a part of your life forever. You wouldn't forget to eat or brush your teeth. Think of your fitness in the same way!

If you need some motivation beyond your personal health to get moving, perhaps the desire to enjoy your children or grandchildren for many healthful years will be a source of

---

Marjorie, a dear friend of mine who just happens to be eighty-nine years old, sent me this exercise recommendation for seniors. I hope you find it helpful:

Senior Exercise

For those of us getting along in years, here is a little secret for building arm and shoulder muscles. You'll find that doing this exercise three days per week is quite effective. Follow the directions precisely for best results:

1. Begin by standing with a five-pound potato sack in each hand.
2. Extend your arms straight out to your sides at shoulder height as long as you can.
3. After a few weeks, move up to ten-pound potato sacks.
4. Over time, work up until you get to fifty-pound potato sacks.
5. Finally, build up to where you can lift a hundred-pound potato sack in each hand.
6. Hold your arms straight out for a full minute.
7. Now, the next step is to start putting a few potatoes in the sacks.
8. Be careful; don't overdo it!

---

motivation. My friend Melody began her lifestyle journey a couple years ago. She wanted to start losing weight and getting healthier so she would be around to watch her beautiful little granddaughters grow up and get married some day. This is what she shared with me recently:

> I'd reached a point in my mid-fifties where I was feeling decidedly "old." I had a total hysterectomy and an old back injury was starting to talk to me a bit more loudly than it used to. I didn't like how old I was feeling, but I tried to convince myself it was normal. But it just didn't feel that way. One day I was playing with my granddaughters and realized that if someone yelled, "Gramma! Go long!" I couldn't do it. I couldn't even follow them around the zoo for the afternoon any longer.
>
> A year later and thirty-five pounds lighter, I'm a new person. I discovered that it does matter what you eat and how much you exercise. Little things do make a big difference. I began to exercise daily, eat less fat, drink more water, and eat more whole foods. Today, I feel ten years younger than the last time we went to the zoo. In fact, my (younger) husband has trouble keeping up with me! I realized that I do have control over things like "aging" and that I can make myself much more productive and energized. It's not about losing weight any longer, it's about maximizing my energy, giving myself endurance and flexibility that I haven't had for years. And using my body feels absolutely terrific!

By understanding how your body works and what you need to be fit for life, I hope you will realize that lifetime fitness is much easier than you may think. A multitude of exercise programs are available in illustrated books, video programs, and at local gyms and health clubs. Explore your local resources to find a program that meets your personal and financial needs. Exercise professionals (such as certified trainers or group class instructors) and professional videos can demonstrate proper form and help you make corrections in your technique when you are first getting started.

If you are battling excess weight, knowing that your body burns fat best during aerobic activity should motivate you to move more. For those of you who love food and want to be lean without dieting, the truth is simple: you must become more active and purposely move most days for the rest of your life.

Don't let that scare you. You don't have to become a fitness fanatic. But increasing your daily activity and active calorie burn is essential. I do believe in the value and long-term benefit of exercise. However, I do know people who have lean, healthy bodies and never break a sweat—they simply lead very active lifestyles and walk almost everywhere they go.

Keeping Yourself on Track

Once you make the decision to adopt a more active lifestyle, the rubber needs to meet the road . . . that is, you need to *do* something. Here are a few ideas that will assist you in your fitness quest:

1. Establish realistic goals.
2. Use a log to track your progress.
3. Reward yourself when you accomplish a goal.
4. Tailor your program to your needs, lifestyle, and physical ability.
5. Be flexible and realistic.
6. Fight boredom during exercise with diversions like music and television.
7. Develop a network of workout partners.
8. Get the green light from your doctor!

Before starting an exercise program, it's wise to get a medical checkup in order to avoid aggravating any existing conditions such as heart disease, high blood pressure, or back problems. If you're over forty or have an ongoing physical condition or other limitation, definitely see your physician.

Total Fitness

There are three components of overall fitness: (1) strength and toning; (2) aerobic endurance; and (3) flexibility. By understanding the role each component plays, you can design your own active lifestyle and become a calorie-burning machine. Whether you choose to join a gym, get a personal trainer, or just engage in fun activities on a regular basis, you will have the knowledge to fine-tune your fitness to meet your personal goals.

1. Strength and Toning

Did you know that your muscles are your body's engine? They burn calories not only during physical activity but also when your body is at rest. Increasing your muscle mass will increase your body's capacity to burn calories. One pound of fat burns only about 3 calories per day. But one pound of muscle burns up to 50 calories. If you gain two pounds of muscle over the next year and nothing else changes, you could lose about ten pounds of body fat.

The good news: Some studies show that exercise can increase your resting metabolic rate by up to 20 percent. In addition, fat-releasing enzymes are manufactured in muscle cells. The more fit and toned your muscles are, the more effective they are at releasing those fat-releasing enzymes. It has been proven that diets, which significantly restrict your caloric intake, can cause the loss of lean muscle mass. Strength training will help you maintain your lean muscle mass while you lose fat and is excellent for toning and shaping the body and preventing injuries. It also helps the following conditions: osteoporosis, arthritis, obesity, aging, hypertension, and high cholesterol.

The bad news: From the age of about thirty on, we begin to lose muscle mass at the rate of up to 10 percent per decade. That means by the time we reach sixty, we've lost as much as 30 percent. In terms of metabolism alone, that could equate to hundreds of calories per day not burned. That, coupled with decreased strength, tone, and support to your skeletal system equates to a weak, unfit, accident-prone woman. Don't let yourself go. Every year (actually every day) makes a difference in your vitality tomorrow.

To build strength, a muscle must be overloaded or worked beyond its normal level. This overloading challenges your muscles on a regular basis and stimulates them to build stronger and tighter muscle fibers. This is best accomplished through some form of resistance training. You can use free weights, machines, exercise bands, or even your own body weight. You do not have to join a gym. There are many simple exercises you can do in your own home using inexpensive equipment and your own body weight for resistance.

Strength training does not necessarily mean you will build large muscles. First, your flabby, untrained muscles will actually get tighter and take up less space. Then, depending on your body type, level of resistance, and frequency of workouts, you may begin to see an increase in size. Women, by nature of their hormones, rarely build large muscles.

You are in control of your results based on your objectives. Muscle tissue actually begins to atrophy within forty-eight to seventy-two hours. If you feel too bulky, just reduce the frequency and intensity of your workouts. Your muscles will begin to shrink without consistent stimulation. But they will *never* turn to fat. And fat cannot turn into muscle no matter how hard you work out. Fat is fat and muscle is muscle!

If your body still has a fat layer over the muscle, you will not see the benefit of all your work initially. However, beneath the surface important things are happening. Your increased metabolism and fat-releasing enzymes will increase the "melt rate" of fat from your body. You will be seeing some of those toned and fit muscles showing under your skin before you know it.

Before you pick up one weight or start getting to work on your trouble spots, it's important to understand that there is no such thing as "spot reducing." Most people are unhappy with the fat that is lying on top of the muscle. For many women, it may be the legs or hips. You may feel compelled to do lots of leg exercises or sit-ups. Those exercises are fine for the muscles, but no matter how many times you "kick" or "crunch," the fat is just going for a ride! If you want to see your toned muscles, you have to lose the excess fat that is lying on top . . . through aerobic activity.

2. Aerobic Endurance

The list of benefits from aerobic exercise seems almost endless. Aerobic exercise has been linked to the prevention of most diseases and even plays a key role in diminishing chronic depression and pain. And one great benefit we all know about is that fat burns best during aerobic activity.

Aerobic means to use oxygen. When we engage in large-muscle, sustained activity such as walking, biking, swimming, or even dancing, we significantly increase the amount of fat being burned for fuel. Large-muscle, sustained activities are considered aerobic because we can maintain them for long periods of time without running out of oxygen. When the activity is isolated to a single muscle group as in weight lifting, or when we exercise so hard we become winded, that is considered anaerobic, or without oxygen.

Aerobic endurance is a measure of how fit your heart and lungs are. Aerobic exercise causes you to breathe more rapidly and your heart to pump faster. With regularity, your body will respond with a lower body fat, heart rate, cholesterol level, and blood pressure. Another positive benefit will be increased energy and endurance. To improve cardiovascular fitness you must engage in aerobic activity for at least twenty minutes, three times per week. That is the bare minimum. Most people need to move more than that to maintain a lean body.

Aerobic exercise elevates your metabolism while you are exercising and keeps it elevated for some time afterwards. The level of "after burn" is dependent on the duration and intensity of the exercise. Aerobic exercise also stimulates other systems in your body that burn calories. The percentage of fat burned for energy steadily increases from about 5 percent fat and 95 percent carbohydrates to over 50 percent fat and 50 percent carbohydrates in the first thirty minutes of aerobic activity. This 50/50 ratio continues from the thirty-minute point throughout the aerobic workout. It's easy to see the most efficient and healthy way to access stored body fat is through frequent aerobic exercise!

Certain types of aerobic activity are more effective than others for weight control. You should pursue those that put the least stress on your body. You may have heard these referred to as non-impact or low-impact. Examples of non-impact aerobic activities are swimming, bicycling, and rowing. Low-impact aerobic activities include step aerobics, aerobic dance, and walking.

I'm guessing that after you read chapter 16 ("What's Your Wheelchair?"), you will celebrate the simple blessing of walking with renewed appreciation. You already know that walking is the easiest, most convenient and inexpensive way to get regular exercise, but I bet you didn't know that walking a mile burns just as many calories as running a mile. That's right. So why run? You get there faster! However, there are far fewer injuries with walking. Because it is low impact, you need little or no stretching unless your muscles feel tight. Here are a few ideas for working more walking into your daily life:

1. Schedule walking meetings. Carry a pad and pen and jot down thoughts you need to remember.
2. Consider your dog's health. He (or she) needs to stay fit too!
3. Pace when you are waiting for someone instead of sitting.
4. Consider walks with friends to catch up on news (rather than meeting for coffee or lunch).
5. Get a good cell phone plan and return all your calls while you walk . . . this one is *my* favorite!
6. Every time you can move, do; it adds up!
7. Make appointments with yourself to walk (and keep them).

Periodically, take short power bursts, picking up your pace, pumping your arms, and going for it until you feel slightly winded. Then slow down and repeat a little later. This will build your capacity to take in oxygen more effectively and gently improve your leg strength as well. Start adding a few hills for more of a challenge. You will be amazed. Within a couple weeks, those hills will be so much easier!

Participating in regular weight-bearing exercises stimulates your body to build stronger bones. Why? Because the regular "pavement pounding" tells your body to get ready for more, and it prepares you by giving you more of what you need—stronger bones and bigger muscles. Pretty cool, eh? Use the muscles, bones, cardiovascular system, and lungs God gave you by developing an active, vibrant lifestyle. It will energize and mobilize your body to become all it was designed to be. Or simply sink into an increasingly sedentary lifestyle and watch your body transform into a living, breathing marshmallow.

3. Flexibility

I don't know about you, but the older I get, the more stiff and achy I get as well. The benefits of stretching and keeping every joint mobile are crucial in these menopause years. Though your flexibility naturally decreases with age, with a regular stretching program, you can slow down the process significantly.

Muscular flexibility improves your posture, appearance, and overall performance. By staying flexible, you will decrease the risk of joint injuries and muscle strains. When you have engaged in too much activity, stretching can help reduce muscle soreness. It is important to stretch properly to avoid injury. Ballistic (or bouncing) stretching is not recommended. Static stretching that holds the muscle in one position without bouncing is best. Stretching is more effective when you warm up first. Warm muscles will relax and lengthen much more readily.

Stretching is both relaxing and invigorating. Instead of just sitting when you watch television, get on the floor and stretch at the same time. If you do this several times each week, you'll be quite amazed at how much better your body feels.

Cross training refers to a training technique that varies the type and intensity of your exercise. There are several advantages. First, the variety allows you to use a wider range of muscle groups. This will enhance overall fitness. Second, cross training will help prevent overuse injuries that result from doing the same thing over and over. Last, it stimulates your metabolism. Your body is an incredibly adaptable machine. If you keep doing exactly the same thing (such as walking or running each day), over time your body will burn approximately 25 percent less calories at that activity. (For those of us who are trying to burn maximum calories, this is not good news.) So, if you walk every day, add an occasional exercise class or bike ride. If all you do is swim, add walking to your routine. Get creative and mix it up; you'll be more fit and lean!

Danna's TV Workout

After more than twenty years of teaching group aerobic classes at athletic clubs and gyms, I was ready to "do my own thing." The music and group energy had served its purpose to keep me motivated for years; but I decided I needed a more time-efficient exercise plan. I realized that by the time I packed up my gym bag, jumped into the car, and drove back and forth to the gym, I could have a decent workout done, so I started to work out at home more often than not. And my most important piece of exercise equipment became my television remote control! That is, I do 90 percent of my exercise while channel-surfing all the early morning news and talk shows. They are a great distraction from my workout and keep me informed as to what's going on in the world.

The Warm-Up

Even though I'm "doing my own thing," it's still important to start with a warm-up. I begin by simply moving around the house, going up and down the stairs, making the bed—whatever gets my circulation pumping. If I'm ready to "jump in" right after "jumping out" of bed, I warm up by walking in place until I feel my muscles loosening up. If any muscle group (especially my legs) feels tight, I do specific stretches for those areas.

The Aerobic Phase

With "clicker" in hand, I'm ready to burn some calories. Ideally, I like to burn 400 to 500 calories before I jump into the shower. I've used a Caltrac Activity Monitor[1] for years to tell me exactly how many I burn. I find it highly motivating and accurate.

Without a monitor, you can simply use a clock and decide how long you want to work out aerobically. I recommend a minimum of fifteen minutes. Once you've built up your endurance, thirty or more minutes will help you maximize the fat-burning benefit of your workout.

Depending on your fitness level, you can walk or jog in place, step side-to-side, alternate high knee lifts, or perform any other type of aerobic move you've learned. Be careful not to be too repetitive, especially when first starting out. It is very important to vary your movement to avoid overuse injuries. Pay special attention to the tightness of your muscles the next day and stretch accordingly.

Another low-impact option is to use a portable step. If you are exercising on a hard surface, use only low-impact moves. That means one foot is always on the ground and you are avoiding a lot of bouncy moves. Highly padded carpeting can be a problem. While it may seem that the extra cushion is good, you can suffer injuries because of the lack of stability and how your body lands on that type of surface. Shoes are just as important in this type of workout as they are if you go out and jog around the block, so put them on and replace them regularly.

Tone and Stretch

It is also fun to do light conditioning exercises using hand weights while you watch your favorite program. Imagine if you committed to doing at least five minutes of sit-ups and a few leg exercises every time you watch television in the evening. Wow. It's so easy and effective. Your clothes would fit better in no time, and you wouldn't feel guilty being a couch potato!

Once or twice a week, have an extra long stretch session in front of the TV. Start at your neck and work your way to your feet, stretching every muscle group along the way. You will feel both relaxed and invigorated in the process. And it is a great way to prevent injury and diminish stress.

For me, combining television with my workout makes the time fly, and I don't feel guilty wasting time "vegging" in front of the tube. Even when I'm exhausted at the end of a hard day, I sometimes forgo the aerobic workout and simply stretch or do some light floor exercises while I watch a favorite program.

Another positive variation is to combine your floor exercise time with catch-up time with family members. The key is to find enjoyable, time-efficient ways to work fitness into your lifestyle.

More Fitness Info

An Ounce of Prevention

There is nothing more frustrating than getting injured once you begin to enjoy the benefits of your fitness investment. Start slow and listen to your body. The old motto "No Pain, No Gain" is a fallacy. Protect yourself from injury by including a warm-up, cool-down and stretch segment in every workout. Additional stretching and a day off should be included any time you feel significant muscular tightness.

Cardiac Alert!

The greatest risk of cardiac arrest is not during intense exercise but at its conclusion. Your body must make major adjustments as your heart rate slows and circulation changes. Always take at least three to five minutes to walk slowly or march in place at the end of an aerobic workout. Check with your physician if you notice any shortness of breath, chest pain, or pressure in your chest. *Don't ignore your body's messages!* It is better to be safe than sorry.

HEALTH FLASH
TIPS FOR HOLY HOTTIES

Get Your Lifestyle into the Act

Even when life gets the best of you and you don't make the time to get a "real" workout, you can find creative ways to get your lifestyle into the act. Here are a few ideas:

- Use the stairs instead of the elevator.
- Get rid of the TV remote control.
- Park at the back of the parking lot.
- Take a walk on your lunch break.
- Take walking visits with your friends.
- Have walking meetings whenever possible.
- Pace when you have to wait for someone.
- Do gardening or yard work.

- Clean up the garage! (At least you'll burn calories!)
- Play ball with the kids or the dog.
- Take active outings like trips to the zoo.
- The list goes on and on!

To achieve total fitness you need a combination of strength, aerobic endurance, and flexibility activities woven into your lifestyle. With consistency, you will start to notice changes in how your body looks and feels. You should begin to feel invigorated and refreshed. Each day you will feel stronger and more energetic.

9

Does Menopause = Fat?

The excessive lifestyles most Americans indulge in can be seen in our rapidly increasing waistlines. The obesity epidemic is flowing across our country faster than melted butter. Is it the food industry's fault that we are fat? While they don't help the problem, they are not its source. As adults, we must take full responsibility for every bite we put into our mouths.

Test your "weight gain" savvy by writing true or false after each of these statements:

1. Women gain weight as they age, regardless of lifestyle.
2. The weight gain associated with synthetic hormones is due primarily to water retention.
3. Diminished thyroid function is often a consideration as we age.
4. If you're fat already, you'll always be fat.

Here are the answers:

1. *False.* The biggest reason that women gain weight as they age is due to the fact I mentioned earlier—decreasing muscle mass. If you can maintain your muscle mass, you will not only burn more calories, you will look and feel much better.

Another interesting consideration is mounting evidence that a lifestyle of reduced calories (30 to 40 percent fewer than the average American diet—which is too high anyway) can actually prevent muscle loss in aging adults. Even more profound is the reality that low caloric intake is the *only* scientifically proven way to increase life span. Some experts say that by decreasing intake by 30 percent, we can increase our life span by 30 percent.[1] That means the average life span of about seventy-five years could be extended to about ninety-seven years.

2. *True.* One of the side effects of synthetic hormones is water retention. There is also a possible correlation to increased appetite. The latter is a matter of choosing not to give in to the cravings. The former can be remedied by using herbal formulas or natural hormones, which tend to have fewer side effects.

3. *True.* Many women have diminished thyroid function, which does not show up on standard blood tests and can be a contributor in middle-age weight gain. For best results, have a saliva test taken. Natural thyroid hormone is a healthier alternative to synthetic. (See further information about thyroid function at the end of this chapter.)

4. *False.* While it's harder to lose weight in the midst of menopause, it can be done. Body fat will diminish if you adopt consistent lifestyle changes, the most important of which is burning more calories than you eat each day.

Counting Calories

No one enjoys counting calories, but the truth is that your body is the perfect calorie-counting machine. Whether you know what you are eating or not, your body does and it always bases its storage and burning of fat on truth. In this chapter, I have taken some of my teaching from my *Scale Down* book to help you deal with the issue of excess body fat. Dealing with bondage to food, emotional eating, and all the spiritual and physical strategies for losing weight permanently are covered in great detail in *Scale Down*. However, if you are simply putting on a few extra "menopause" pounds (especially around the middle), I think you will find these fat-burning basics quite helpful.

Here is a well known statistic: The average woman gains about twenty-five pounds between the ages of twenty and fifty. How many extra calories do you think she needs to eat for this to occur? You may be surprised. It is only about 5 calories! That's the equivalent of one breath mint a day.

If you keep eating exactly what you're eating and only add that one mint per day for the next thirty years, you'll gain about twenty-five pounds! Sounds like really bad news, doesn't it? But the opposite is true also. If you burn 5 calories more a day than you eat, you'll lose twenty-five pounds over thirty years. But who wants to wait that long?

If we take the same principle and simply multiply it, we can accelerate the process. For example: If you burn 100 calories more than you eat per day, you'll lose ten pounds in a year doing nothing different. Now let's work both sides of the "energy equation," both intake and output. If you eat 100 calories less and burn 100 calories more, you have a difference of 200 calories each day. That's twenty pounds in a year. The point is that little stuff adds up. It's like money in the bank gaining interest. At first, you don't think your little lifestyle changes

are making any difference because you don't see any indica-
tion on the scale. It's still happening. We just don't realize
that those small shifts in our eating and moving really add
up. People can move from a two-story house to a single level
and gain ten pounds simply because they're not running up
and down the stairs every day burning calories!

Your Body—An Energy Bank

As far as I am concerned there is nothing new under the
sun when it comes to weight loss. True experts concur over
and over despite the weight loss hype that the bottom line in
losing excess weight is simply calories in versus calories out.
I know that doesn't sound very sexy, but it's the truth. Our
body is an energy bank; it stores and releases energy based
on deposits and withdrawals. Most of us are making too many
deposits and not enough withdrawals. This is just the opposite
of what we are often doing in our financial lives. If we could
reverse the two, we'd be on the right track—physically and
financially!

I'd like to illustrate why understanding your calorie bank
account is so important. Let's assume I gave you a checkbook with $2,000.00 in it and sent you off to the mall. In
this wonderful imaginary exercise, I'll give you two hours to
spend it all. Wow, what fun! But, I have a couple important
rules: (1) You cannot subtract one single purchase until you
are all done; and (2) If you go over by even $1.00, you owe
me $2,000.00.

Most of us would fail miserably because we are not good at
accurately assessing what we are spending (or eating). When
we go to a bulk food store, we usually make the most of each
trip. At the checkout, the overflowing cart tells us it's going to
be an expensive purchase. However, we still aren't prepared
for the grand total when it comes. The same thing happens

when we first get a job and start paying our own bills. We are surprised at how little we have left when the last one has been paid. This is also the case as it relates to our body's calorie bank account.

The Bottom Line to Your Bottom Line

Our body is a perfect calorie-counting machine; it is absolutely accurate. When someone says, "I don't know what went wrong. I've gained twenty pounds over the last year," I can tell you exactly what went wrong. You ate more calories than you burned. Now, in menopause, those extra pounds will have a tendency to collect around the middle, especially if you are taking estrogen and not absorbing it effectively. (See chapter 11 for more information on that very important subject.)

A very small percent of the population has a metabolic challenge. And for those who do, it's rarely the whole issue. The bottom line is that the body counts every calorie. If you eat more than you burn, the body will store the excess calories as fat. Again, it is important to note that as we age, the tendency to have an underactive thyroid (which may not show up on a traditional blood test) may also play a role.

When people say they lost weight on this or that diet, the primary reason for the loss is a caloric shift. Whether it's the Submarine Sandwich Diet, the Hollywood Diet, the Blood Type Diet, the Atkins, or the Ronald McDonald Diet, weight is lost because you burn more calories than you eat. Statistics show that over 90 percent of people who lose weight on a diet gain it all back (and usually more) within a year. My advice is simple: stop dieting. (If you want to explore these issues in depth to include the mental, emotional, and spiritual aspects of weight loss, I suggest you read my book, *Scale Down*.) I dieted for almost sixteen years without finding any permanent answers. Then I discovered a powerful truth secondary only to renewing my mind as detailed in chapter 4. Here is my weight loss philosophy in a nutshell:

> You need to lose weight the same way you plan to keep it off. The only way to do that for a lifetime is through a lifestyle change. When making lifestyle changes, ask yourself this question: "Can I maintain this way of eating, exercising, and living most days for the rest of my life and still enjoy my life?" If the answer is "no," you're probably on another diet or extreme exercise program. If the answer is "yes!" you've made a lifestyle change.

Today, the average American woman burns about 1,700 calories per day. At the turn of the century, she probably burned closer to 2,500 per day. That's a huge difference. Why? Her lifestyle was much more physically demanding. Our automated, sedentary lifestyles are dramatically different. We need to simulate activity (move and exercise purposely to get that kind of calorie burn). Most people are not moving enough for good health, let alone burning all the calories they eat.

For the last decade I've used the Caltrac Activity Monitor to tell me how many calories I burn all day long. Based on my age, height, weight, and sex, it calculates my resting metabolic rate (the number of calories I burn laying flat for 24 hours) and my moving calories (the number I burn in my daily activities). As a 52-year-old, 5'7", 140-pound woman, I burn about 1,400 calories laying flat for 24 hours. If I just go through my normal day without purposeful activity, I burn another 300 calories for a total of about 1,700 calories. But you know what I found out? My appetite is about 2,000 calories per day. So if I eat 2,000 and only burn 1,700 calories, those extra 300 calories are being stored as fat on my body. Bummer.

Making Small Changes

With a very simple equation and very modest lifestyle changes, you can burn off one pound a week without ever dieting. Here are the facts: There are 3,500 calories in one pound of fat. So if you burn 500 calories more than you eat every day, you will lose one pound of fat each week. I recommend doing this as a combination of increasing output (calories burned) and decreasing intake (calories eaten). That's a lifestyle change. Try to find small ways to eat less and move more every day. You will be absolutely amazed at what happens over time. By the way, the scale is definitely *not* the way to measure this loss.

My client Kathy was a great example of applying simple changes to realize profound change. In analyzing her lifestyle habits, we discovered two important issues. First, she was drinking at least three regular colas (nearly 350 calories) a day. In addition, she rarely exercised. Over the course of three months, Kathy only had two to three colas per week and started walking a mile and a half each day. She lost about thirty pounds and kept it off!

The point is this: find creative ways to modify your eating and activity permanently. If you try something too dramatic, you probably won't stick with it. But small changes that don't seem too difficult will add up if you practice them consistently: stay off the scale; measure your success by your behavior and by how your clothes fit over time; and, most important, change your behavior internally by changing the way you think about food. Apply the principles in chapter 4 ("The 'Change' That Transforms Your Life") and you will have no more need for willpower. If you truly believe you can eat and live healthfully and know what that means, your behavior will eventually follow.

I Really Can't Lose Weight!

If you are certain you are doing all the "right" things but are still struggling to get the fat off, you may be one of the 25 percent of women who have "Syndrome X." These women are extremely insulin sensitive. That is, whenever they eat easily digested carbohydrates, their body shoots out insulin and converts those carbohydrate calories into stored fat. These people need to be very careful about eating high fiber and protein with every meal and snack. By the way, most women who don't have Syndrome X would also benefit from diminishing processed carbohydrates as much as possible.

Another factor that makes it more difficult to lose weight is stress. Stress makes us fat in several ways. Although the behavioral response to stress is often thought to be a primary reason for weight gain (for example, we reach for ice cream when we feel stressed out), there are two very powerful physiological reasons for the link between stress and weight gain. First, whenever we are under stress, our bodies release the stress hormone known as cortisol. In the body, cortisol is a potent signal to do two things—increase appetite and store fat. Second, cortisol partnered with the other primary stress hormone, adrenaline, triggers a release of glucose into the blood stream. Because we rarely engage in physical activity when we are stressed, the excess sugar, if not burned off, can create dangerous side effects such as those of diabetes. Therefore, the hormone insulin is immediately excreted to transport the sugar to fat cells. This stress cycle happens day after day in the lives of many women.

In small amounts, cortisol is needed by the body to control carbohydrate metabolism, inflammation, and cardiovascular function. While small amounts of cortisol are a "good" thing, too much cortisol, for too long, is most certainly a "bad" thing because it leads to the development of a number of adverse health conditions such as diabetes and depression.

Within our fast-paced modern world one might ask: "Who doesn't have elevated cortisol levels?" Dozens of scientific studies on cortisol reveal that the following three groups of people are highly likely to suffer from elevated cortisol levels:

1. Those who experience daily stress (work deadlines, family demands, bills, traffic).
2. People who get less than eight hours of sleep each night.
3. Chronic dieters who restrict calories for weight loss and dieting or have restrained eating habits.

Unfortunately, diet supplements are not magic. You will still need to address your stress issue and eat properly to lose weight. You'll do well (and save money) by not investing in every diet aid that hits the market.

Change That Lasts

If you want to make a change that lasts, you need to find ways to modify your lifestyle that you can live with. There are many misconceptions about losing weight. The oldest is that you have to diet or make some drastic change to actually lose weight permanently. Think about your first diet. How old were you? What kind of diets have you tried? How many worked? If this has been an ongoing struggle in your life with issues of emotional eating and chronic dieting, I encourage you to read my book *Scale Down*, which deals with this challenge in depth, helping you make permanent change from the inside out.

Why not make a decision to surrender this issue of your body and habits once and for all to God? In the process, give yourself permission to be human and strive to follow these checkpoints toward lifestyle victory:

- I am finding creative ways to eat fewer calories every day.
- I am finding simple ways to burn more calories every day.
- I am learning to eat for maximum energy and health.
- I am making purposeful activity or exercise a regular habit.
- I am identifying and changing my unhealthy beliefs and attitudes.
- I am building a foundation of truth from God's Word to live victoriously.
- I am becoming transformed by the renewing of my mind.
- I am learning to see myself and my goals through God's eyes.

I think we agree that there are no quick fixes. Seek truth and take the small steps that will permanently change your body. Those small steps become your new lifestyle . . . something you can live with and even enjoy. That will make the changes in your body and attitude permanent. And isn't that worth the investment?

HEALTH FLASH
TIPS FOR HOLY HOTTIES

Thyroid News You Can Use

When you're hypothyroid, you don't feel well! If you are experiencing weight gain without overeating, hair loss, fatigue, low libido, high cholesterol, dry skin, low basal temperature—or any of dozens of other unresolved symptoms that drastically affect your quality of life—your symptoms may be thyroid related. Some hypothyroid patients also suffer from muscle pain, lethargy, and depression. The treatment may include natural hormone therapy, nutritional supplementation, and changes in diet and lifestyle.

According to pharmacist Amanda Edelman, an expert in naturally compounded hormone therapy with Life Wellness Pharmacy, more than 20 million people in the U.S. suffer from thyroid disease. Among these are 10 million women with low or borderline-low thyroid levels. More than 30 percent of women over fifty suffer from low thyroid symptoms. But many are never accurately diagnosed due to the inadequacy of blood serum testing methods.

Almost all forms of thyroid disease lead to a single outcome: the condition of hypothyroidism—an under-active, under-functioning thyroid gland. If left untreated the symptoms can be physically, mentally, or emotionally challenging.

Do any of these symptoms sound familiar?

Gaining weight without overeating

Persistent fatigue or exhaustion

Irritability

Frequently feeling cold

Unexplained depression or anxiety

Mental fogginess

Dry skin or hair

Low libido

Sleep difficulties

Unexplainable aches and pains

Blood Serum Testing

If you answered yes to one or more of the symptoms above, you should consider having your thyroid tested. But all testing is not equal. According to Ms. Edelman, standard serum thyroid tests measure overall levels of specific thyroid factors, not the factors that are truly available to the body. Unfortunately, most medical clinicians use blood serum testing for thyroid function as their primary diagnostic tool regardless of the accuracy. These tests can often yield a "normal" test result because of the wide range that is considered "normal." Yet the individual is truly deficient in "active" thyroid factors. Perhaps you have been told by your medical clinician that your thyroid test is in the normal range, but you wonder why you feel so poorly. If the symptoms above persist without relief, you should pursue a more accurate (and less utilized) method of testing.

Saliva Testing

Saliva testing measures *only* the free or available thyroid hormones in the body—those that can be utilized readily. This type of testing is much more sensitive to detecting low or insufficient levels of thyroid hormones. You must be your own health-care advocate and insist on saliva testing. Companies such as Life Wellness Pharmacy in Carlsbad, California, will send you a saliva kit that you can use in the privacy of your own home. After the results come in, they will consult with you personally over the phone and interface with your physician to determine if natural, bio-identical thyroid hormone replacement is needed. Just as synthetic estrogen is difficult for the body to effectively assimilate, synthetic thyroid is inferior to its natural counterpart.

The Ultimate Test

The greatest test of all is how you feel. If a blood test indicates normal thyroid levels but you still exhibit symptoms, a low dosage trial of a thyroid medication might be a consideration.

Menopause symptoms such as hot flashes, night sweats, and weight gain, and many other types of medical conditions can be much more pronounced than low thyroid levels. Energy levels, quality of sleep, and stamina are directly affected by thyroid levels.

Taking Action

1. What was the most important truth you gained from this chapter?
2. What changes, if any, do you desire to make related to that truth?
3. What specific thoughts or actions need to be implemented to make those changes?
4. What are your greatest stumbling blocks toward this change?
5. On a scale from one to ten (with ten being the highest) how important is this relative to other needs/changes in your life? Use this scale to help you create an overall action plan when you finish reading this book.

10

The ABCs of Lifestyle Change

In the previous three chapters, we reviewed the most essential "basics" to living a healthy lifestyle. Most of us, however, don't implement what we know to be good for us because we operate using faulty belief systems. Without the right attitude, belief, and consistency of action, nothing will happen. In chapter 4, I discussed how to be truly transformed by the renewing of your mind.

Of course, we always need to look to God's Word to validate what those attitudes and beliefs should be. If they aren't in sync with his truth, replace them! It is also appropriate to create healthier messages specific to your personal issues or habits. For example, if you feel compulsive about eating every time you sit down to watch television, you can give yourself a new message: *When I sit down to watch television, I don't feel like eating.* If you tell yourself that message long enough, you will start to change your thinking. That is a simple biological truth about how God designed your brain. In the meantime, tune in to your attitudes and internal messages. They may be leading you down a frustrating, even destructive path.

Harmful Attitudes

In the area of lifestyle change, many of us need to throw out our past attitudes and embrace healthier perspectives. Explore some of the common mental stumbling blocks that follow and make an effort to replace them with healthy, new attitudes.

The "All or Nothing" Attitude

Do you think of yourself as either "on" or "off" some sort of lifestyle program, exercise regime, or diet? That kind of "all or nothing" thinking says nothing counts unless you're doing it "all the way." Nothing is further from the truth in living a healthy lifestyle. Everything counts. And it's the small stuff day after day that will make the biggest difference.

Don't worry about tomorrow or even the next hour. Just live in the moment and surrender it to God. When you blow it, move on. Don't give up and stay stuck. You know that God forgives us when we sin; receive that forgiveness. (And please don't overspiritualize every lack of perfection. We need to honor him with a balanced and healthy perspective as well as a healthy body. Perfect lifestyles require way too much time and attention to the physical body. Good moderate, consistent habits and attitudes will produce the best results.)

Think of your lifestyle journey as a less than direct route toward your destination. Imagine walking across a room by taking three steps forward and two steps back over and over again. Don't focus too much on the two steps back. Focus on the three steps forward and celebrate the fact that you *are* making progress.

The "Quit Before You Start" Attitude

Do you always end up quitting before you start because you have failed so many times in the past? This destructive thinking has grown out of years of failure. Stop allowing yourself to wallow in past failure and draw a line in the sand, step over it, and make a fresh start today. Begin celebrating every little success as a small deposit in your future. If this has been your attitude for some time, I know that the spiritual truths we'll explore in this book will be of great encouragement. Besides, you're reading this book, so you've already "begun" . . . why not continue?

The "Quick Fix" Attitude

Let's say it together with conviction: there are no quick fixes—despite what all the weight loss products promise. Even the most exciting new discoveries usually come with great risk. Remember Phen-Fen? Fortunately, the Federal Trade Commission is really cracking down on outrageous claims and advertising, so fewer people are getting duped. But, don't we all wish that just one of these weight loss or anti-aging wonders were the real McCoy?

There is a prevalent attitude especially in the area of weight loss that demands a painless, no effort, fast, and lasting solution to our fat storage problems. We seem to think if we can get the weight off *fast* we will somehow miraculously possess the inner strength, motivation, and know-how to keep it off. This is the biggest lie. The only things shrinking in America from this attitude are our wallets. The next time you're tempted to buy "Exercise in a Bottle" or "The Ultimate Fat Burner," resist.

143

Many of these products seem to give improvement simply because you *believe* they will. Scientists have consistently found that 30 to 40 percent of all patients given placebos show improvement for a wide variety of symptoms. Placebos work if the person believes they should. This provides fascinating proof of how the mind and body work together!

The "It's Not My Fault" Attitude

"There are always tons of goodies at my workplace." "My friends are always asking me out to lunch." "My life is too busy to fit in exercise." "It's way too hard to shop and cook healthfully." This attitude blames everyone but the real culprits, you and me! Get rid of this attitude and excuse once and for all. Besides, all excuses are equal, and they are all equally worthless.

Perhaps you have a thyroid problem. Take your medication and realize that your lifestyle is a much bigger influence on your weight than your slightly diminished thyroid function. Perhaps you come from a family of overweight people. If you do the right things with consistency, you won't be like them. You may not be the leanest creature on the planet, but you won't be the fattest either! No one shoves food down your throat or forces you to live a sedentary lifestyle. Take responsibility and stop letting others influence your choices.

The "I Don't Have Time" Attitude

For years I used to say, "There's not enough time in the day!" How arrogant that I thought God had designed the calendar wrong. The problem was my priorities and expectations. One great equalizer in life is time. The days we live have all been given an equal allotment: we share the same sixty minutes of each hour and the same twenty-four hours of each day. The difference is in how we choose to invest our time. It's been said that we make time for whatever we decide is most important. For most of us, time does not get easier to manage. Short of retirement or death, it will always be a matter of choice. Choose to be the master of your time and find small, consistent ways to invest in your lifestyle daily. If you wait until tomorrow, it will never come. Before you know it, it's too late.

A Healthy Attitude

A healthy attitude is one that finds a balance between current pleasure and future benefit. It allows freedom for flexibility and occasional indulgences without sacrificing health and well-ness. A healthy attitude says, "It's my body and my choice. I'm choosing this because it is important and if I neglect myself too long, I will pay the price."

If you need a little more motivation for making some positive changes in your eating and weight, here's a powerful little fact that could dramatically extend your life. In *The Hope of Living Long and Well*, Dr. Francisco Contreras states that eating a very nutritious diet of 30 percent fewer calories can add 30 percent more time to your life span, in addition to supercharging your overall health.[1] That means if you expect to live to the average age of seventy-five years, you can increase that amount to ninety-seven and a half years just by eating less. In fact, he states that *eating less is the only proven method to increase longevity*.

In the Health Flash on the next page, you will have an opportunity to evaluate your lifestyle in several categories and design a plan to build a healthier body.

One hot-flash sister wrote about lifestyle and menopause and made me laugh out loud. She said: "Midlife means that you become more reflective. . . . You start pondering the 'big' questions. What is life? Why am I here? How much Healthy Choice ice cream can I eat before it's no longer a healthy choice?"

Today is a new day and a fresh start. Let's purpose to find *solutions*, not excuses. It doesn't matter what challenges are holding you back. If you want to achieve victory, you *must* find ways over those speed bumps.

HEALTH FLASH
TIPS FOR HOLY HOTTIES

Four Lifestyle Evaluations

Trying to begin new lifestyle changes without a good evaluation is like letting a dentist drill on your teeth before he takes X-rays! Without a plan, you are destined to fail.

Ignorance is not bliss! If you don't know what the problem is, you can't fix it. It's time to be totally honest; excuses and rationalizations undermine your achievement. Only the truth will set you free. Begin by taking these self-evaluations. They will give you a good snapshot of your current strengths and weaknesses in four categories that will impact your lifestyle and health: (1) perspective/motivation; (2) nutrition; (3) fitness; and (4) fat management. You don't have to take a lot of time. Just determine two or three things in each category that are the most important. Start there and add more when you are ready.

Spend about four to five minutes on each evaluation. Base your answers on your most consistent behavior or attitudes in the past three months. Don't rate yourself based on any changes you've made in the last four to six weeks; rate yourself based on your first impression and move on. Don't go back and readjust your answers if you don't like the score! Remember: this is a reality check. Just face the truth and move on. Now it's time to face the music. Grab a pencil and be completely honest. No one has to see the results but you.

Lifestyle Evaluation—Perspective/Motivation

Based on the last three months, please rate yourself as:

> **0 = Almost Never**
> **1 = Sometimes**
> **2 = Often**
> **3 = Always**

_____ I see myself as a fully accepted and loved child of God.

_____ My choices and actions are made based on my relationship to Christ.

_____ I am thankful for the body God has given me.

_____ I honor God with my lifestyle habits.

_____ I take responsibility for my body's size, shape, and health.

_____ My attitude is this: I am not my behavior. I am complete in Christ.

_____ I surrender my weaknesses to God and rely on his strength for the moment.

_____ My personal goals are realistic and honor God.

_____ I take realistic steps toward my goals each day.

_____ I know that with God's help, I can have a lean, healthy body.

_____ I am aware of the lies I believe about my body, looks, and health.

_____ I recognize and choose not to accept this negative thinking.

_____ I renew my mind with God's truth each day.

_____ I am a work in progress, and God delights in each good step I take.

_____ I choose to submit my body, mind, and spirit to God.

_____ I pray for power to walk in the Spirit and not fulfill the desires of my flesh.

Add the total of all scores.

Scoring:

40–48	Excellent! You have a godly perspective.
31–39	Good. Your perspective is usually working for you.
22–30	Fair. It's time to get a new focus—truth.
< 21	Alert! Alert! Change your perspective now.

Lifestyle Evaluation—Nutrition

Based on the last three months, please rate yourself as:

> **0 = Never or "Don't Know"**
> **1 = Sometimes**
> **2 = Often**
> **3 = Always**

_____ I think about what I eat and how it impacts my health.

_____ I have high energy to do all the things I want and need to do.

_____ I read labels and choose many foods based on that information.

_____ I eat two to three servings of fruit each day.

_____ I eat three to four servings of vegetables each day.

_____ I choose whole-grain products over more processed foods.

_____ I know how much fiber I'm eating daily.

_____ I drink ten to twelve glasses of water daily.

_____ I eat breakfast every day.

_____ I eat a good source of protein at breakfast.

_____ I eat lean protein with my lunch.

_____ I limit my "empty" calories to less than 15 percent of my total diet.

_____ I limit caffeine and other stimulants, such as over-the-counter diet aids, especially those containing ephedra and ma huang.

_____ I take a multivitamin supplement daily.

_____ I take an antioxidant supplement daily.

_____ I choose "healthy" fats in my diet like olive or canola oil.

Add the total of all scores.

Scoring:

40–48 Excellent. Your body loves you.

31–39 Good. You're on the right track.

22–30 Fair. It's time to try a little more high octane fuel.

< 21 Poor. Your body's crying "Help!"

Lifestyle Evaluation—Fitness

Based on the last three months, please rate yourself as:

> **0 = Almost Never**
> **1 = Sometimes**
> **2 = Often**
> **3 = Always**

_____ I crave activity and find ways to move more each day.

_____ I enjoy exercise and how it makes my body feel.

_____ I have high energy to do all the things I want and need to do.

_____ I make exercise and activity a priority in my life.

_____ I understand the need for aerobic, strength, and flexibility training.

_____ I engage in aerobic activity four or more times per week.

_____ I take the stairs or park far from my destination whenever I can.

_____ I monitor my heart rate and know I am exercising safely.

_____ I am injury-free and able to engage in most activities freely.

_____ Being healthy and fit is important to me.

_____ I listen to my body and know what it needs.

_____ I wear appropriate and quality shoes for exercise.

_____ I have a very active life and am moving throughout the day.

_____ I work out my major muscle groups two to three times each week.

_____ I can easily touch my toes without bending my knees.

_____ I maintain strong abdominal muscles.

Add the total of all scores.

Scoring:
40–48   Excellent. You're a fit machine.
31–39   Good. Stay consistent.
22–30   Fair. Use it or lose it.
< 21   Poor. Take one small step and start moving!

Lifestyle Evaluation—Fat Management

Based on the past three months, please rate yourself as:

> **0 = Almost Never**
> **1 = Sometimes**
> **2 = Often**
> **3 = Always**

____ I feel in control of my food choices.

____ I measure my size by how I look and feel, not the scale.

____ I eat only when I'm hungry.

____ I stop eating when I'm full.

____ I understand why "calories count."

____ I eat four to five small meals or snacks per day.

____ I limit my junk food, fast food, and desserts to less than 15 percent of my diet.

____ I am happy with my body weight.

____ I am happy with my size and shape.

____ I can enjoy "fun food" without feeling guilty.

____ I think about food only when I'm hungry.

____ I can see myself eating and living in control.

____ I walk or get purposeful exercise at least four times per week.

____ I am very aware of my choices and how they affect my body.

____ I say no to the latest diets or supplements promising quick results.

____ I know that if I'm going to be lean, I have to take daily action.

Add the total of all scores.

Scoring:

40–48	Excellent. You've got a lean lifestyle.
31–39	Good. You're doing most things right.
22–30	Fair. It's time to take action.
< 21	Poor. Start with one step at a time.

11

HRT—Yes or No?

News flash! Menopause is *not* a disease. This is how Webster's Dictionary defines it: "the natural cessation of menstruation." Does that sound like a disease? It is expected. It is natural. And it happens to every woman blessed to live that long. As Dr. Stengler writes in *Your Menopause, Your Menotype*, "Women don't need a cure; they need guidance and relief. Just because you remedy symptoms with a drug doesn't mean you've effectively and healthfully addressed the problem."[1]

There are many physical and emotional challenges associated with menopause, but that doesn't mean you're sick. The purpose of this chapter is to address the issue of hormone replacement (both synthetic and natural) in generalities so you are equipped to research and determine what is best for *you*. Keep in mind, your decision today may change in a few months or years. That is why you need to be well educated about how to best care for your body.

I'll be candid from the outset; based on personal research and extensive consultations with noted health experts, I am opposed to synthetic hormones. I believe there is a more effective and safe alternative. Don't just accept my take on this; research for yourself and decide what is best for you.

Estrogen

Let's take a look at hormone levels and how we can find balance as naturally as possible. As Dr. Stengler states:

> It's inaccurate and much too simplistic to say that menopause is caused by an estrogen deficiency alone. In fact, progesterone levels drop and other hormones also fluctuate dramatically. As we age, our bodies metabolize hormones less effectively. This may be one way God naturally protects us since elevated hormones pose a greater risk of uterine and breast cancer. Just having low hormone levels does not mean that you absolutely need hormone replacement therapy.[2]

God designed this, ladies. When you begin to run out of eggs, your hormone levels begin adjusting. Unless you have severe symptoms or a major risk factor such as osteoporosis, there's really no reason to put extra hormones into your system. Only significant deficiencies coupled with problematic symptoms or risk factors warrant hormone replacement therapy.

Synthetic HRT

Feminine Forever, written by gynecologist Robert Wilson, hit the market in 1966 and promoted the idea of synthetic hormone replacement as the magic pill that would restore a woman's "femininity" and maintain her youth. *Feminine Forever* was distributed by pharmaceutical sales reps to doc-

154

I think I was about seven years old when the now famous fashion doll Barbie hit the market. I loved my Barbie. I assumed that when I became a teenager, I'd have long, thin legs, a trim waist, and nice perky breasts just like her. (Little did I know that most females with long, thin legs only have nice "Barbie" breasts if theirs are plastic just like hers! That's because the body type that gets thin legs doesn't get large breasts as well. I guess it's God's way of being "fair.") Well, Barbie turned fifty in 2009 and is approaching menopause quickly. I heard that someone is thinking up some special new Barbie models. Perhaps if they ever hit the market, they will help our granddaughters relate to their red-hot grandmas! Here are a few possibilities I received via email:

Hot Flash Barbie

If you press her belly button, you can watch her face turn beet red while tiny drops of perspiration appear on her forehead. She comes with a handheld fan and tiny tissues.

Facial Hair Barbie

As her hormone levels shift, you can see her little chin whiskers grow. Also available: teensy tweezers and a magnifying mirror.

Flabby Arms Barbie

She's got the flap-in-the-wind triceps that swing to and fro as she brushes her hair and little dumbbells to help her fight the flab.

Postmenopausal Barbie

This Barbie wets her pants when she sneezes, forgets where she puts things, and cries a lot. She comes with her own supply of Depends and Kleenex.

tors' offices all over the country, and excerpts from the book appeared in many women's magazines. By 1975, more than six million American women were taking Premarin. This hormone replacement therapy is better known these days as "HRT." By 1999, an estimated fifteen million women had prescriptions for hormones.[3]

Our generation was not the first to identify the benefits of hormone replacement. Ancient Chinese texts describe elders who rejuvenated their sex lives by drinking the urine of teen-aged boys and girls. (The urine contains hormones.) Another form of hormone therapy was adding the placenta of a newborn to soup or making it into pills. I know it sounds disgusting, but science followed the same example. The most widely prescribed hormone in the world—Premarin—comes from the urine of pregnant horses. Thus the name, clearly abbreviated from "*pre*gnant *mare* ur*ine*." How natural!

Synthetic hormone products come in limited dosages; women get to choose only from what is manufactured for the masses, not necessarily what their bodies need. Just imagine going to a department store and having only sizes four, ten, and sixteen to choose from when shopping for a pair of jeans. None of those sizes fit me! It seems the pharmaceutical industry cares more about a patent and maintaining marketing exclusivity than their desire to help women in the most beneficial way.

Until recently, most conventional doctors suggested synthetic hormones the first time their patients reported a hot flash or missed period. According to registered compounding pharmacist Michael Lenzner, over eight million women in the United States are on some form of synthetic hormone therapy to help alleviate symptoms associated with menopause. (It's no wonder, since half of the adult women in America are in some stage of menopause.) However, when the landmark 161,000-woman Women's Health Initiative study on synthetic hormone replacement was abruptly halted in July of 2002, shock waves reverberated through the medical community. The National Institutes of Health (NIH) cancelled the fifteen-year study ten years early because they felt the increased health risks of synthetic hormone replacement outweighed the benefits. The study was on combined estrogen plus progestin—the most commonly used treatment by menopausal women who have not had a hysterectomy. The data revealed that "women on HRT had more invasive breast cancers, heart disease, strokes and blood clots. The study's positive findings—a reduction in hip fractures and colorectal cancer—did not outweigh the added harm."[4]

Doctors and patients became confused about how to respond. A large percentage of women stopped taking hormones cold turkey without even consulting their doctors. Some doctors instructed their patients to cease taking their hormones, expressing uncertainty about long-term side effects (not to mention the potential liability). Two years later, however, it is estimated that more than half the women who stopped HRT out of fear returned to synthetic hormones when their unmanageable menopausal symptoms returned in full force.

The federally funded Women's Health Initiative also enrolled about eleven thousand women in an estrogen-only study, but, at the time of this writing, a second bombshell in its long-awaited review of hormone therapy has been dropped. The NIH has prematurely stopped the study after seven years "in the interest of safety of the study participants." The NIH believes that, based on the data so far, "estrogen does not provide the reduction in heart disease that was anticipated and hoped for. Indeed, estrogen therapy is apparently increasing some health risks, especially the risk for stroke."[5] With about eight and a half million women using some type of synthetic hormone therapy and the vast majority on estrogen only (not estrogen plus progestin), the results of the estrogen-only trial are exceedingly relevant. To date, the findings translate to about sixty-eight hundred excess strokes per year among postmenopausal women. Other studies reveal a trend toward increased risk of cognitive impairment and dementia.

Please note that the Women's Health Initiative used synthetic, not natural, hormones. Synthetic hormones are branded and patented pharmaceutical drugs. Patents allow drug manufacturers to price, sell, and market their prescriptions as unique creations. To obtain a patent for a synthetic hormone (or any other drug), the molecular structure must be modified. The result is a hormone that looks very similar to a natural hormone but is very different in structure and function.

You may wonder why pharmaceutical companies have never taken a look at herbal and natural remedies, including natural hormones. As Dr. Stengler writes:

> The economics of the pharmaceutical industry make such a research investment impossible. No one can patent a food substance found in nature. Without a patent, a company cannot corner the market on a product and control its price. So even if a natural product is safer and more effective than a prescription drug, no pharmaceutical company has an incentive to promote it.[6]

Natural HRT

There are alternatives to synthetic HRT. Many health-care professionals, including Dr. Stengler, suggest these choices: First, make purposeful lifestyle changes such as the nutrition, exercise, and stress reduction changes we've already addressed in previous chapters. These will help support your body's natural inclination to seek balance. Second, try natural remedies to address the untoward symptoms of menopause as mentioned in the Health Flash regarding black cohosh in chapter 1. Then, if you're still not getting adequate relief, discuss a season of natural prescription hormone therapy with your personal physician if an accurate analysis of your hormone levels warrants it. At times, that is the only thing that will adequately address persistent night sweats, hot flashes, and, most importantly, advanced osteoporosis. Unlike branded drugs, natural prescription hormones cannot be patented (because they have not been corrupted). They are compounded to have the same molecular structure and function to those naturally occurring in the body.

Natural HRT is a reasonable alternative to synthetic HRT. Also called "bio-identical" hormones, they are indistinguishable in molecular structure and function to those found naturally produced in the body. They are derived from plants such as soy, wild Mexican yam, and other natural sources. It is thought that by mimicking nature, these compounds, which are native to our bodies, will provide relief from menopausal symptoms without the level of risk associated with synthetic hormones. Many ancillary, anecdotal studies point in that direction. Unfortunately, there is no big study like the Women's Health Initiative in progress, since no financial motivation exists to explore this alternative in depth.

Natural hormones are available by prescription from specialized compounding pharmacies and cannot be purchased over the counter. Dr. Stengler recommends a conservative approach to natural HRT. His philosophy is this: "Take the lowest dose of natural hormones for the shortest duration possible to avoid any potential untoward effects." This strategy includes regular saliva hormone tests to accurately evaluate your body's response to therapy.

A Difficult Choice

Because my mother had breast cancer, I had concluded I would *never* mess with any type of hormone replacement. No symptom would be worth the risk. As they say, "Never say 'never'!" First, I was not well informed about natural hormone replacement options. Second, when I made that exclamation I'd never experienced unrelenting, insomnia-producing, bed-soaking night sweats. After months of averaging four hours of sleep per night and finding little relief from herbal and other remedies, I asked Dr. Stengler to write me a custom compounded prescription for natural HRT. The relief came rather quickly. My husband was even more pleased than I. I was nicer to be with both day and night!

> This winter I did something I said I would never do. I bought an artificial Christmas tree. It looked so realistic I could hardly tell it was man-made. I guess the fact that the needles stayed green and fresh looking for more than a week was a dead giveaway. Every real tree I've purchased over the past few years died days before Christmas! My advice is this: go artificial on trees ... and natural on hormones!

I kind of missed my hot flashes this winter when I stayed at our mountain cabin. But blankets and cozy fires are a lot easier to deal with than a body that has no responsive thermostat. As my girlfriend's adult children used to ask, "Is it hot in here, or is it just Mom?"

You holy hotties know exactly what it's like to have your own private summer in the middle of January, don't you? Taking hormones of any kind requires serious consideration and the help of a trusted health-care professional who is not afraid to seek the most natural approach available.

According to pharmacist Michael Lenzner, founder of Life Wellness Pharmacy in Carlsbad, California, synthetic hormones are still prescribed by most doctors and may be appropriate in some instances, but they are only an appropriate choice if both the patient and physician are fully educated on alternatives.

After several months of steady hormones, I slowly weaned myself off the natural hormones and tried one of Dr. Stengler's therapeutic herbal formulas. I am pleased to say that today I am staying about 90 percent symptom-free with this herbal approach. I plan to have a comprehensive hormone test every twelve to twenty-four months, depending on my symptoms, so I can stay at the top of my game.

HEALTH FLASH
TIPS FOR HOLY HOTTIES

Hormone Testing

Saliva Testing

Saliva testing is the most reliable way to measure the hormones that are actually doing their job at the cellular level. Most blood tests do not measure these "bio-available" hormone levels. In addition, saliva testing more accurately reflects tissue uptake and the response of hormones delivered topically (through the skin), in creams, gels, or patches. This type of testing has been used scientifically for decades and has been shown to be highly accurate. The World Health Organization uses this method of hormone testing in worldwide comparisons of breast cancer among women living in industrialized and nonindustrialized countries.

According to Dr. Stengler, several other reputable studies have validated this form of testing as the most accurate and dependable. You can do this in the privacy of your own home, collecting multiple samples throughout the day or week to ensure a more comprehensive analysis over a "one shot" blood draw. Make sure to use well-known companies and work with a knowledgeable doctor to help you interpret the results if you do the testing at home. Dr. Stengler feels that saliva testing will probably become the most popular method of choice in the next several years. Saliva hormone testing kits are available from holistic doctors, health food stores, and pharmacies specializing in custom compounded natural hormones.

Note: Women on hormone therapy will have altered saliva hormone results, which must be taken into consideration when analyzing the results.

Other Methods

Urine testing is another way to measure hormone levels. Some researchers feel it is more accurate because of the various samples collected over a twenty-four-hour time frame.

While blood tests may be less accurate in measuring active hormones, they are the only way to measure levels of 16 alpha-hydroxyestrogen, a metabolite associated with breast cancer risk.

If you are experiencing menopause symptoms and want to address your issues most effectively, get a hormone test that includes not only estrogen and progesterone but testosterone, DHEA (the anti-aging hormone), and thyroid. This is the best way to ensure you are addressing your issues at the root cause.

Taking Action

1. What was the most important truth you gained from this chapter?
2. What changes, if any, do you desire to make related to that truth?
3. What specific thoughts or actions need to be implemented to make those changes?

4. What are your greatest stumbling blocks toward this change?
5. On a scale from one to ten (with ten being the highest) how important is this relative to other needs/changes in your life? Use this scale to help you create an overall action plan when you finish reading this book.

12

Hormone Hostage Husbands, Part One

Puppies are the most wonderful little creatures. They are so cute and cuddly (until they piddle on your carpet, chew up your favorite shoes, get muddy paw prints on the beige sofa, and shed little hairs all over your white slacks). My favorite puppy, Widget, grew into a beautiful, shiny, black cocker spaniel.

I should have been paying closer attention twelve years ago when Widget had her first litter. I had no idea that how she handled her mate, Gizmo, would be a "prophecy" for my husband, Lew. Poor Gizmo . . . poor Lew.

Throughout the animal kingdom, there are sad victims of females' "raging hormones." I call those victims "Hormone Hostage Husbands" or "HHHs."

From early pregnancy on, Widget lost all patience with Gizmo. She would not let him eat next to her from his own bowl as he had for many years. Every time he approached, she would snarl until he cowered away. He couldn't curl up and sleep close to her. He couldn't play with any of their toys, because whatever Gizmo happened to have in his mouth Widget wanted, and she wanted it now!

The ultimate insult came after the puppies were born. We created a nice little "nursery" in the garage where Mom, Dad, and puppies could bond and live without making a mess of my house. There was plenty of room for all eight members of the furry family to coexist. Apparently Widget didn't agree. When Gizmo approached the puppies, she growled like a wolf. When he walked toward his bed, she almost bit his head off. If he approached the water dish, she went chasing after him. Confused, shaken, and clearly defeated, he often retreated to the farthest point of the garage and, with his nose firmly planted in the corner, stood there completely still for over ten minutes until Widget fell asleep nursing her pups. Poor hormone hostage doggie!

Through the years, when I would get a little "edgy" and hormonal, Lew would occasionally try to get me to lighten up by standing "nose to corner" to make a point. We'd chuckle and I'd get the message.

However, I never anticipated that I would *become* Widget. At the height of my menopause madness, I not only wanted Lew's "nose in the corner," I sometimes wanted him out of my sight completely. Poor guy. No matter what he did, it irritated me. When he snacked on something crunchy in the bedroom at night, I'd cringe; each bite sounded as if he were dancing on gravel with metal shoes. Some days he would stroke my arm as we relaxed on the sofa watching TV, and I would get incredibly irritated. It felt as if a bug were crawling on my skin. "Do you *have* to do that?" I'd ask with obvious exasperation. He'd look at me as if to say, "Where's my wife and how did Cruella De Vil invade her body without my noticing?" (I later found out in my research that this "bug crawling" feeling on the skin is a common complaint of many women during menopause. I hate bugs.)

Communication Is the Key

From pregnancy to PMS to menopause, every HHH knows that there are days when all he has to do is open his mouth and he takes his life in his hands. Let's face it: there are some questions men should *never* ask. An unknown source once shared the following handy tips to help men avoid becoming a casualty of raging hormones. Pass them on to your man to help him avoid those awkward "HHH" moments.

Dangerous: What's for dinner?
Safer: Can I help you with dinner?
Safest: Where would you like to go for dinner?

Dangerous: Are you wearing THAT?
Safer: Gee, you look good in brown.
Safest: Wow! Look at you!

Dangerous: What are you so worked up about?
Safer: Could we be overreacting?
Safest: Here's fifty dollars.

Dangerous: Should you be eating that?
Safer: These apples are so delicious!
Safest: Are you craving chocolate, honey?

Dangerous: What did you DO all day?
Safer: I hope you didn't overdo today.
Safest: I've always loved you in that robe.

Yes, those husbands who learn quickly how to "manage" menopause madness have a much easier road.

An article titled "The Good Wife's Guide" in *Housekeeping Monthly* in May of 1955 gave tips for how to greet and treat your husband at the end of a hard day's work. I've rewritten and summarized them.

If you're feeling a little hormonal as you read this chapter, fasten your seat belt . . . this may put you over the top. But before you blow a gasket, please note that I have provided a corresponding tip for your guy as his "Good Husband's Guide to Surviving Menopause."

Good Wives—Tip #1

Have dinner ready. Plan ahead, even the night before, to have a delicious meal ready, on time, for his return. This is a way of letting him know that you have been thinking about him and are concerned about his needs.

Good Husbands—Tip #1

Call her midafternoon to see what kind of food she's in the mood for tonight. Then find out if she'd like takeout or would prefer to dine at the restaurant. Be ready for last-minute changes; respond with great flexibility. How you handle her whims will determine the quality of *your* evening.

Good Wives—Tip #2

Prepare yourself. Take a fifteen-minute rest so you'll be refreshed when he arrives. Touch up your makeup and put a ribbon in your hair and be fresh looking. He has just been with a lot of work-weary people.

Good Husbands—Tip #2

As the Bible says, "Gird up your loins." Be ready for any-thing the night may deliver. Come through the door ready for action. And she really doesn't care how you look, just so you don't look critically at her!

Good Wives—Tip #3

Be a little exuberant and a bit more interesting for him. His boring day may need a lift and one of your duties is to provide it.

Good Husbands—Tip #3

Be a little invisible. Until you ascertain her mood, don't express much emotion. And by all means, *don't* come home with another menopause joke. She's not laughing. Only *women* are allowed to tell menopause jokes.

Good Wives—Tip #4

Clear away the clutter. Make one last trip through the main part of the house just before your husband arrives.

Good Husbands—Tip #4

Hire your wife a good housekeeper.

Good Wives—Tip #5

Minimize all clamor. At the time of his arrival eliminate all noise of the washer, dryer, or vacuum. Try to encourage the children to be quiet. Arrange his pillow and offer to take off his shoes. Speak in a low, soothing, and pleasant voice.

Good Husbands—Tip #5

Minimize every possible sound. At the time of her arrival reduce all noise of the lawn mower, sports channels, or any power tools. Try to encourage the children, pets, and even the neighbors to be quiet. Arrange her pillows and offer to take off her shoes. If you must speak, do so in a low, soothing, and pleasant voice with as few words as possible.

Sometimes we need to "turn the tables" to better understand what our spouse's life is really like. Whether you are a domestic engineer or work full-time outside the home, it's hard to fully comprehend what stresses and challenges your mate may endure. Even in the midst of your most intense menopause madness, pray for the strength and grace to be the "good wife" God has called you to be for your husband.

The grass is not greener on the other side of the fence; it's just different. Despite the challenges of being a woman, including the pain of childbirth and the irritations of menopause, I've never wanted to be a man. I appreciate the unique ways God has created us. No matter what you think you are going through, never forget that your Hormone Hostage Husband is surfing the meno-waves too, as the tides of your hormones and emotions rise and fall.

God's Plan for Marriage

I have heard several accounts of marriages that crumbled to pieces in the "heat" of menopause madness. I think we should honestly scrutinize anything that is diminishing the quality of our marriages. Menopausal or not, we must invest huge energy into this most important of sacred institutions. It is the oldest establishment sanctioned by God and essential to the healthy survival of any society. Let's take a look at God's ultimate plan and our responsibility as daughters of the King.

In the Beginning

Did you ever notice how many times in Genesis 1 it says "God saw that it was good" after an aspect of his creation? The first time God says something negative about creation is in Genesis 2:18: "It is not good for the man to be alone; I will make him a helper suitable for him."

One man I heard about was sick and tired of his lot in life. His wife was a homemaker and he went to work every day convinced that she had a much easier life than he. He wanted her to better understand the load he was bearing and so he prayed:

"Dear Lord, I go to work every day and put in eight hours while my wife merely stays at home. I want her to know what I go through, so please create a trade in our bodies so she can understand."

So God, in his infinite wisdom, did just that. The next morning when the man awoke, sure enough, he was a woman. "He" arose, cooked breakfast for his mate, awakened their kids, set out their school clothes, fed them breakfast, packed their lunches, drove them to school, picked up the dry cleaning, stopped at the bank, paid all the bills, and went to the grocery store, all before 1:00 p.m.

Then he cleaned the litter box, bathed the dog, made the beds, did the laundry, vacuumed, dusted, and mopped the kitchen floor before running back to school to pick up the kids who argued with "him" all the way home. He set out a nutritious snack and got them organized to do their homework and then set up the ironing board close by to lend assistance as necessary.

At 4:30 p.m. he began to peel the potatoes, wash the salad greens, snap the fresh beans, and bread the chops for supper. After a wonderful meal, he did the dishes, folded the laundry, bathed the children, and put them to bed.

At 9:30 p.m. he was exhausted and though his chores weren't done, he went to bed where he was "expected" to make love to his relaxing "husband"—which he did without complaint.

The next morning he awoke and immediately knelt by the bed and prayed, "Lord, I don't know what I was thinking. I was so wrong to envy my wife's role in this family. Please, Lord, let us trade back!"

The Lord replied, "My son, I feel you have learned your lesson and I will be happy to change things back to the way they were. You'll have to wait nine months, though. You got pregnant last night!"

What an incredible Creator we have; he loves us completely and designs us for intimate connection with him and with each other. The power of authentic intimacy is almost indescribable.

We cannot thrive fully without it. The most important of our human relationships is, of course, our marriage. Its quality will impact our lives profoundly—especially during difficult times. If your marriage has an unshakable foundation, praise God! Pass on the wisdom you have gained to all the women in your life, because even in Christian circles, marriages are crumbling at an alarming rate.

I've heard it said that we are drawn to and fall in love with those who make us feel good about ourselves. Why then at this stage of life do so many women feel poorly about themselves and apathetic at best about their marriages?

During this time of "change," you may be more insecure and vulnerable than ever. Perhaps you are questioning your outward beauty or your value to others. Go back to all you know to be true. Go back to memories of how and why you and your husband fell in love. Most important, go back to the source of all love—God.

Two Shall Become One

After God declared that Adam indeed needed a partner, he caused a deep sleep to fall upon him. God took one of Adam's ribs and "fashioned into a woman the rib which He had taken from the man, and brought her to the man. The man said, 'This is now bone of my bones, and flesh of my flesh; she shall be called Woman, because she was taken out of Man.' For this reason a man shall leave his father and his mother, and be joined to his wife; and they shall become one flesh" (Gen. 2:22–24).

My pastor and radio partner, Dr. Tim Scott, thinks that in most men there is both an emotional and spiritual striving to become whole based on God's original design to create them with a need for a helpmate. In essence, Dr. Scott believes that man is incomplete until he becomes one with a

171

lifetime mate. At a recent wedding, Tim told the new couple they were acquiring a new identity that day. He was not referring to the identity they already had in Christ but to the new distinctiveness that bonded them together as one flesh . . . soul mates for life. This is the ultimate and perfect union our Creator had in mind. Of course, that was before sin entered the picture.

Whether you are in your first marriage or fifth, God's ideal right now is for you to have perfect oneness, first with him and then with your spouse. You cannot undo the past, but you can be renewed for the future. As believers living in a fallen world, we are waging war against the enemy and even against our humanistic society that says difficult relationships should be discarded and replaced. This lie tells us there is no hope. This lie says nothing can make things right again. Take those lies and discard them; replace them with truth. With God, all things are possible. Let's take a closer look at love and discover how we can become the helpmates God has truly called us to be.

Motivated by Love

If you've ever fallen deeply in love, you know that your mind is flooded with almost obsessive thoughts about that person. You reflect on your moments together and wonder what he is doing and thinking right now. You write your name next to his . . . then your name with his last name (you *know* that you did!). You anticipate your next encounter with great expectation. Every little thing you can do to make his life easier is your greatest joy without a thought about how it might inconvenience you. It seems in the early stages of love that many men and women can actually live out the words so beautifully penned by the apostle Paul in 1 Corinthians 13:4–7:

Love is patient, love is kind and is not jealous; love does not brag and is not arrogant, does not act unbecomingly; it does not seek its own, is not provoked, does not take into account a wrong suffered, does not rejoice in unrighteousness, but rejoices with the truth; bears all things, believes all things, hopes all things, endures all things.

The purest of love is all those things. It truly empowers us to be the loving creatures God intended us to be. It gives us a sense of significance, value, and purpose. This kind of love is a driving force and motivation behind all we desire. The love Paul speaks of is agape love—a selfless pouring out of ourselves for other people, not only our soul mate.

Yet why does the intensity of love often stale and our motivation to please those we care about wane? What has changed? Is it us . . . or is it love? I suspect that what really changes is our perspective. Over time, we see our husband with eyes of familiarity. That in itself is not a bad thing. But with familiarity, we also have a tendency to see our mate's flaws more vividly than his virtues. When left unchecked or coupled with other circumstances, we may also begin to view him with eyes of discontent, criticism, or disrespect. Our relationship is in dangerous waters, and we must recognize the relational shipwreck on the horizon if negative attitudes aren't nipped in the bud.

Think back to the man you fell in love with years ago. Is he really that different at his core? I suppose, like you, he still has many of the same dreams or desires. And, like you, over the years, he has experienced his share of disappointment—disappointment in others (including you) and mostly in himself. His "first love" attitude has also run a bit dry and with it the self-propelled motivation to speak your love language.

The sad fact is that while women are dealing with the biggest transitions of life (menopause, empty nest, and an aging body), many husbands may be in the throes of a midlife crisis. That, coupled with "familiarity disease," may explode into marital disaster. No matter how much you and your husband love God, you are in vulnerable times. Be wise; ask the Lord to help you see, understand, and empathize with your husband's life season. Pray that he will open the eyes of your heart and ignite your love in fresh ways.

I love the wise words shared in Pam and Bill Farrel's book *Marriage in the Whirlwind*. Quoting their mentors, Jim and Sally Conway, regarding how a wife should view her husband in this "mid-life era," they write: "He wants his wife to be a girlfriend and a lover, not just a mother and a household manager. 'Be your husband's best friend. Understand what he's going through and attempt to meet his needs. In other words be fun and sexy, not naggy or bossy.'"[1]

They go on to write how Sally dealt with Jim's crisis. She says, "I began to think in terms of how a younger woman would act around him. I decided to look at him with the eyes of a twenty-two-year-old and tell him what I saw in him and how I felt about him. I wanted to affirm him more and act more flirtatious."[2]

The point is this: the vitality of your marriage in the best years of your life (the ones you have left) will depend largely on how you choose to see and respond to your husband. Men grow increasingly sensitive as they age; this may be due in part to their decreasing testosterone and increasing estrogen levels. (Yes, they have both!) But, just as likely, they learn over the years the value of connectedness. If you model connection that is fueled by the kind of passion you had when you met, your man will likely melt over time.

Don't wait for your husband to respond according to your expectations before pulling out all the stops to invest in a marriage that will endure the decades to come. Love as you know he wants or needs to be loved and leave the rest to God. The enemy would confound you with lies saying that your husband's actions are evidence that he doesn't deserve your love and devotion. That may be true. But we don't deserve the abundant grace and love Christ has bestowed on us. If he waited until we deserved it, we'd all perish in hell!

Love is the essence of our life in Christ. We find lasting satisfaction despite our circumstances when we fully embrace divine love (vertically) and then extend it (horizontally) to our earthly relationships. Mature, abiding love will sustain us and we in turn will help sustain others down the most difficult roads of life.

You will find blessing and satisfaction when you love "as unto the Lord" despite your mate's response. Jesus, your "perfect husband," will fill in the gaps where all human men will fail. Let those disappointments go and celebrate the gift God has given you.

People change most when they are loved consistently and unconditionally. We all desire it. But few of us give it unless there is reciprocity in our relationship.

If you are living a one-sided relationship with a selfish or withdrawn husband, love him anyway. And if for some reason he never responds, run to the arms of your heavenly Father. (A few godly girlfriends are blessings from heaven as well!)

When asked what was the greatest commandment of all, Jesus replied, "'You shall love the Lord your God with all your heart, and with all your soul, and with all your mind.' This is the great and foremost commandment. The second is like it, 'You shall love your neighbor as yourself.' On these two commandments depend the whole Law and the Prophets" (Matt. 22:37–40).

Did you get that? All the Law and the Prophets depend upon loving God and loving others. Love? That's it? Is it really that simple? Yes, if we focus on this one thing, all the other pieces of the puzzle will fit together. Love is the sustaining glue. This seems easy when we are in the "in love" phase of our relationship. But loving selflessly becomes difficult after years of what my husband calls the "mature love phase." I think a huge part of the problem is that we follow our emotions more readily than our minds. We need to understand abiding and committed love; it may not give us butterflies, but it is solid, warm, and secure.

No matter how old we are, it is human nature to put ourselves first. When people disappoint us, betray us, or leave us, we move into self-protection mode because the center of our universe is self. Even as believers capable of walking in the Spirit, we still can fall into self-absorption and self-protection. To love as God calls us to love, we have to *choose* to look up, surrender our hearts to God. We must be willing to put our hearts "out there" even if it means risking getting hurt.

Too often self-protection results in diminished expressions of "true" love as expressed in 1 Corinthians 13. In fact, without the Spirit of God living in us, we are incapable of real agape love. Our normal mode says, "You love me, I'll love you. You hurt me, I'll hurt you." After years of reactionary loving, our love is no longer expressed in selfless giving.

I'm sure you've noticed that it's easy to get a lot of emotional bumps and bruises on our hearts in the journey to live with Christ at the center of our lives. As young women, we measure our value by who loves us. Later, we may invest much of our self-worth in our children, our work, our ministry. If we place all our needs for love and significance in the hands of mere mortals, material possessions, or accomplishments, we will ultimately be disappointed, even devastated. I know.

I did that once as a very young woman and lost myself for a season. The next time I was betrayed, though my heart was broken, I stood on solid ground and experienced the tangible love of Christ because I knew whose I was despite the rejection from my husband. When we intimately know the author of love, we can love without concern for self-protection.

God's Love for Us

You sang the song as a child . . . or sang it to your children. You certainly believe it for them. But, do you really believe it for *you*? Stop for a moment to digest that simple, yet most profound truth. We exist simply because our Creator chose to give us life. In fact, he is our life-support system. Every single breath we take is because he chooses to give it to us. He loves us beyond our ability to imagine and it is this same love that motivated him to bridge the gap between his perfection and our sin by sacrificing his Son. It is this love that draws us to himself. The Bible says that we love because he first loved us.

When I am struggling with feelings of inadequacy or feeling detached and all alone, I find many areas in Scripture comforting. One of my favorites is Psalm 139. It grounds me in the truth of God's intimate and personal love for me.

> O, Lord, you have searched me and you know me.
> You know when I sit and when I rise;
>> you perceive my thoughts from afar.
> You discern my going out and my lying down;
>> you are familiar with all my ways.
> Before a word is on my tongue
>> you know it completely, O Lord.
> You hem me in—behind and before;

you have laid your hand upon me.
Such knowledge is too wonderful for me,
    too lofty for me to attain. . . .
For you created my inmost being;
    you knit me together in my mother's womb.
I praise you because I am fearfully and wonderfully
    made;
    your works are wonderful,
    I know that full well.
My frame was not hidden from you
    when I was made in the secret place.
When I was woven together in the depths of the earth,
    your eyes saw my unformed body.
All the days ordained for me
    were written in your book
    before one of them came to be.

                       Psalm 139:1–6; 13–16 NIV

We seek intimacy and meaning more often from mere mortals than we do from a perfect God. By reversing our priorities, we make ourselves vulnerable to heartbreak and disappointment. People fail. And then, our sense of significance falters. But when a deep intimacy with God is our first priority, we have a foundation that can never be shaken. Even when the rug of life is pulled out from under us, we have a "solid rock" that keeps us strong—the unconditional love and acceptance of a perfect Father.

If you sense that some of the challenges you are having in your marriage are due to your own insecurities about being worthy or lovable, meditate and pray about these truths. Pray that you will see yourself accurately and love the people in your life as if you'll never get hurt. Even if you do get hurt, there is One who will never leave you or forsake you. His love is sufficient and perfect when all others fail.

The Emotional Bank Account

Years ago, in my corporate days, I facilitated for a Fortune 100 company a program based on Stephen Covey's *The Seven Habits of Highly Effective People*.[3] In it he taught a concept that I have used ever since called "The Emotional Bank Account." It's pretty simple. With respect to our relationships, we need to evaluate if they are in the "black" or the "red" based on emotional deposits or withdrawals. Intimacy will diminish if our account is low or out of balance. Both parties in a friendship or marriage must be making deposits. Then, when one spouse is needy or difficult to deal with, withdrawals will not bankrupt the relationship emotionally.

Every mature partnership realizes that each person may travel through difficult seasons, which requires more grace and mercy in their time of need. But if there is never a time of meaningful deposit, the "grace-giving" partner may grow weary. As believers, we know that we are to have hearts willing to forgive and serve without expectation. We may do that out of obedience and love. And that is good. It is unfair though to expect our partner to simply put up with us out of Christian "duty."

Despite our "power surges" and changing bodies, we need to take responsibility for how we respond to the challenges of menopause. We may feel like screaming, "It's not me; it's my hormones!" but we still must learn how to manage our bodies and our emotions so we don't create undue stress for those who cross our paths. Most of us can maintain our composure at work or in public, but we get to the safety of our homes and, pow! Watch out, family!

The emotional safety provided by those who love us is not an invitation to take advantage of that security. Will they love us if we explode in their faces? Yes. Will they forgive us if we are short-tempered and difficult to live with? Yes. Will they accept us even when we act selfishly or withdraw? Yes. But chances are if we are withdrawing more from them than we are depositing, they will begin to withdraw or avoid us out of self-protection (or simply to maintain their own sanity).

It is human nature to withdraw from pain. We don't leave our hand on a hot stove because we know from experience it will burn us. Most men will self-protect from a hormonally challenged wife after months of being pushed into a corner. It's our job to learn how to cope in ways that don't push those we love too far away. There needs to be a balance of clear communication, effective coping strategies, and a massive dose of grace all around.

I propose that on our "good days" we make an extra effort to deposit into our husband's emotional bank account large donations of what is most important to him! If you don't know it already, discover your husband's "love language" as taught by Gary Chapman in his bestseller, *The Five Love Languages*.[4] Does he respond to acts of service, gifts, positive affirmation, touch, or quality time the most? We often make the mistake of trying to make deposits into another's life based on *our* love language. It will be much more effective to deposit based on *his* specific need.

So, on a scale of one to ten with ten being highest, how is your bank account doing with the most important people in your life? If you are presently married, how is it with your husband? Perhaps a more accurate assessment would be asking *him* to rate it. Then ask him the best way to fill it to the brim.

My husband has been an expert in filling my emotional bank account. Just knowing he understands and tries so hard to give me what I need speaks volumes to me about how much he loves me. And as I find more personal balance and victory in managing this life stage, my heart is filled with a desire to extend both grace and love to him when he goes through work or midlife challenges himself. Although, at this writing I must confess I am still quite overdrawn. I think I've got a few ideas for his bank account this weekend. I'm sure you have some for your hubby too!

HEALTH FLASH
TIPS FOR HOLY HOTTIES

The Power of Authentic Connection

Our mental and relational health has a direct impact on our physical health. Committed relationships make a huge impact in our lives. They are the source of most of our joys *and* sorrows. When life stresses and emotional disconnection wear you down, you become more vulnerable to physical stressors as well. Perhaps this simple "connection" exercise will bring your relational health into greater balance. It has been proven that healthy, authentic relationships (especially with our spouses) have a profound impact on all the dimensions of our lives. Live long, stay connected, and thrive!

Authentic Connection Exercise

These questions are designed for both partners in a relationship (marriage or deep friendship) to evaluate one another's contribution to the relationship in a very transparent way. You must be aware that complete honesty may expose some painful areas in your relationship that will need work. If you have the courage and desire to know what others truly desire from you, give them the freedom to share transparently without fear of hostile confrontation and do the same for them. The best way to respond to their answers is to simply ask questions for clarification. The worst way to respond to any negatives is to defend yourself or attack their weaknesses. Do you have the courage to grow?

1. If you could change one thing about me, what would it be?
2. How would that change impact our relationship?
3. On a scale from one to ten (with ten being the highest), how would you rate our relationship in the following areas:
   a. ____ The amount of time we spend together
   b. ____ How we spend our time
   c. ____ Our ability to communicate
   d. ____ The level at which you feel I understand you
4. Overall, does our relationship energize or drain you?
5. What is your greatest need in our relationship?
   a. How do I meet that need?
   b. How do I miss that need?
6. Do you feel your expectations for our relationship are in sync with mine?

Taking Action

1. What was the most important truth you gained from this chapter?
2. What changes, if any, do you desire to make related to that truth?
3. What specific thoughts or actions need to be implemented to make those changes?
4. What are your greatest stumbling blocks toward this change?
5. On a scale from one to ten (with ten being the highest) how important is this relative to other needs/changes in your life? Use this scale to help you create an overall action plan when you finish reading this book.

13

Hormone Hostage Husbands, Part Two

Years ago, a friend told me that she and her husband had not been sexually intimate for over four months. At the time, I had been married to Lew for about five years and couldn't imagine what could keep two people physically distanced for that period of time. That was "pre-menopause." Today, I better understand both personally and from other mature friends why this is not an abnormal occurrence.

Approximately 80 percent of postmenopausal women experience a significant decrease in libido. According to Dr. Stengler, there are two main causes: physical and relational/emotional factors. Later in this chapter, I'll address the physical factors. For now, let's take a look at the emotional and relational implications.

Emotional/Relational Factors in Intimacy

Many once-demonstrative wives become uncharacteristically disinterested or even repelled by sexual intercourse because of a variety of causes. Despite the "reason" for our decreased libido, husbands can be impacted profoundly by how we respond sexually. While short seasons with diminished intimacy are very normal, it is our responsibility to discover what is causing our low libido and address those issues as best we can.

The emotional/relational side of the equation gets a little complicated. When our relationship with our husband is not strong and vibrant, adding menopause emotions and our own corroding self-image to the mix can be devastating to intimacy.

This one chapter cannot address the full spectrum of possibilities influencing your sex life. I am sure you recognize some of the issues that have negatively influenced your marriage. If you know your union is in danger, run, don't walk, to the best marriage specialist you can find and address those issues now.

Two of my favorite authors who write and counsel extensively on this subject are Bill and Pam Farrel. You will find their bestselling books *Marriage in the Whirlwind*, *Men Are Like Waffles—Women Are Like Spaghetti*, and *Why Men and Women Act the Way They Do!* incredible tools for mending broken relationships. And, of course, quality Christian therapists are magnificent assets *if* you are willing to implement their suggestions.

Relational Disconnection

Cell phones are wonderful, frustrating devices. They connect us to others conveniently and seamlessly at times. Then . . . blip . . . the person on the other end of the phone is gone, leaving you yelling, "Can you hear me now?" We often discover how much we miss our convenient little communication tool when we fail to charge our battery the night before. So it is with our marriages. We have the means to connect, but through glitches in communication or lack of "battery charging" we slowly begin to lose the signal that keeps us connected in true and abiding intimacy.

Have you become disconnected from your HHH due to busyness, unresolved conflict, life pressures, or simply lack of quality time? No matter. The solution is to make your marriage a priority once more. This is a complex issue, but you don't have to understand all the reasons why you're disconnected if you know and practice consistent habits of reconnection. The first of these is obvious—spend more time with each other. The second follows—make it quality time. Talk. Laugh. Share experiences like you did when you first met. Bill and Pam Farrel offer a multitude of suggestions in their book *Men Are Like Waffles—Women Are Like Spaghetti*. Try a few of these ideas to reignite and fan the flame of your love.

> **Look Back**: Try a date that revisits some of those early memories of your life together. Take a trip to the place you first met, first kissed, or where your marriage proposal took place. If finances or distance are a concern, take a picnic together and bring a photo album of the early years and reminisce. Put on "your" song in the stereo and take a drive to your old neighborhood, high school or college, or a favorite restaurant. . . .
>
> **Look Ahead**: Each of us keeps a list of "dream dates" that we'd like to go on. Once a year we remake the list and give it to each other as a "gift." We also give each other a "love list" of at least ten things that are free that make us feel loved. Having these lists helps us surprise one another on a regular basis. By looking ahead you can also plan to invest in your marriage by attending a marriage seminar, conference, or retreat. . . .

When a couple will invest in one another's dreams and plan for the transitions of life, they gain the ability to fall in love over and over again.

Seize the Moment: Invest in the now. Practice the art of touch. Reach over and hold a hand, give a squeeze, pat a back—if you're within arm's distance—try to make contact. With all the technology available today, there are plenty of ways to reach out and touch the one you love. Leave a message on voicemail, fax a love note, email a message that is filled with symbols and word pictures that only you two will understand. Try something radical—stop by home or your spouse's work just to whisper, "I love you"; then drop a single rose on the desk as you leave.[1]

Romance doesn't have to take a lot of money, just a little bit of time spent thinking about your mate. After all, the gift your spouse most enjoys is you!

HER NEEDS

You need to get specific and tell your husband what will build intimacy back into your heart. Let him know what will fill your emotional bank account. Don't buy into the lie that he should "know" without being told. He doesn't. Tell him. But wait! Not so fast. How you tell him is important. Timing and your choice of words are everything. Ask yourself how *you* would want to receive the same information. Be sure the message is positive and not accusatory. Don't use statements such as "You never do this [or that] for me anymore" or "Why don't you ever listen to me? I need you to listen." He may get defensive if he feels he is being criticized or attacked. Tell him first what he already does to fill your bank account; then tell him what you need right now in this stage of life. Take responsibility for your part of the disconnection; then ask him what he needs.

HIS NEEDS

As you know, men are not as verbal as women. Many are very uncomfortable expressing themselves emotionally, but there is something that almost always fills a husband's emotional bank account no matter what his love language may be—sex. Sex makes men feel connected, and they don't have to feel connected *before* sex to have sex (like we do). It's a dilemma we've got to work through. My advice to you is to figure out how *you* can get to the place physically and emotionally where regular, satisfying sex with your husband is something you desire and enjoy.

Statistics show that couples with good sex lives are happier and more likely to stay together (yes, even Christians). That takes me to a slightly touchy subject—your sexuality. If you have "issues" of any type, deal with them. Talk to a counselor or find a mature woman with a very vibrant and healthy marriage and ask for advice. I believe that as women we have great influence in our marriages by how we address this issue. I am not saying that we manipulate our spouses with sex. I am saying that we must get to a healthy place where we can give our bodies to our husbands (even sometimes when it's not on the top of our list) simply out of love.

Thoughts on Intimacy from Scripture

What does the Bible say about sex and marriage and most specifically about times of abstinence in marriage? Not much. There are many references to purity and sexual sin, but what about sex within marriage? First Corinthians 7:3–5 acknowledges our human vulnerabilities when it comes to sex and gives us a godly response to our natural human urges:

The husband must fulfill his duty to his wife, and likewise also the wife to her husband. The wife does not have authority

187

over her own body, but the husband does; and likewise also the husband does not have authority over his own body, but the wife does. Stop depriving one another, except by agreement for a time, so that you may devote yourselves to prayer, and come together again so that Satan will not tempt you because of your lack of self-control.

Once we are married, we are no longer "our own." Just as we become one with God at our spiritual rebirth and are temples of his Holy Spirit, we become one with our husbands in marriage. We need to come to see each other as extensions of our very being. This can be difficult when we are disconnected emotionally. You can see from the passage above that physical deprivation can lead to temptations common to man. While most people think first about issues of infidelity, this is not the only risk to marriages lacking sexual intimacy. The lack of self-control may manifest itself in seeking satisfaction in other ways that diminish the marital bond. For women, this can be close female friendships taking the place of true connection with our spouses. Our girlfriends are incredibly important, but when they distract us from investing in our husbands, we must be very careful.

So does this Scripture passage command us to have sex when we don't really want to? In essence, it does instruct us in being selfless with our bodies. Remember, we *chose* to enter into the covenant of marriage with this man we're lying next to each night. That covenant made us one flesh. A healthy marriage needs sexual intimacy to thrive.

Physical Factors in Intimacy

Without getting graphic, let me say that some sexual intimacy is possible no matter what the physical limitations. Whether your husband is functionally impotent or intercourse is extremely painful for you due to menopausal symptoms, you can still have meaningful erotic connection with your spouse. Now I'm a little old-fashioned and would be too embarrassed to give you specific ideas. Besides, my publisher would probably delete them if I were bold enough to write them down! Seriously, though, there are ways to please each other that don't have to include sexual intercourse.

I have a friend who married a quadriplegic and shared in generalities that they had a very vibrant sex life. How? I'm not sure. What is encouraging is that *they* figured out how to make it happen because they loved each other so much. Renée Bondi (whom I write about in chapter 16) even became pregnant as a quadriplegic.

If we get beyond our parochial hang-ups about sex and realize that our loving Creator designed us as sexual beings, we will have much more satisfying intimacy with our husbands despite our physical limitations. The true objective of sex is not pure physical pleasure but physical union that leads to authentic intimacy only a husband and wife can share.

If you wonder if what I say about God and sexuality is true, take some time to review Song of Solomon. As a brief example, we read in chapter 7, verses 1–3:

> How beautiful are your feet in sandals,
> O prince's daughter!
> The curves of your hips are like jewels,
> The work of the hands of an artist.
> Your navel is like a round goblet
> Which never lacks mixed wine;
> Your belly is like a heap of wheat
> Fenced about with lilies.
> Your two breasts are like two fawns,
> Twins of a gazelle.

Okay, maybe having our navel compared to a goblet doesn't get us all excited, but it is quite sensual to imagine a loving husband adoringly describing his bride from head to toe. He is reveling in her physical beauty and sensuality. What woman wouldn't melt at being celebrated with such abandon? That is what God has designed us for—a deep emotional, physical, and spiritual connection with our husbands.

For the most part, the flavor of your sex life will depend upon your receptivity to your husband's needs and desires. Tell him what you need to feel most connected to him sexually. Most men will have a high motivation to respond to your request. Think about it . . . for them, the reward is what they need to feel connected to you.

Body Image Misconceptions

How we see ourselves (especially as we begin to sag, bag, and drag) has a huge influence on our sexual desire. While most men are easily stimulated by the female body despite its imperfections, women can become so repelled by their own bodies that they cannot become sexually aroused. I covered body image in depth in chapter 3, but let me make a few more comments specific to your sex life.

During sex, most husbands are not focusing on all the things you hate about your body. If you see yourself as the wonderful, sexual creation God made you to be and respond accordingly, your husband will be drawn to you. It is essential that you see yourself accurately through God's eyes, not the world's. Do what you need to feel attractive and sexy, but realize that how you respond and try to meet your husband's needs will draw him more to you than your physical beauty.

Rarely do you hear a man say, "I'm just not comfortable having sex anymore because I look so fat." Men hardly ever

When all is said and done, it is always healthy to maintain a sense of humor. If you and your husband can openly discuss your sexual issues and laugh together through the seasons of life, it will help to take the edge off the intensity of emotions. This "bedroom story" made me laugh.

My husband and I had an evening of intense passion and when I woke up the next day, I couldn't find my estrogen patch anywhere. I changed it as prescribed, twice a week, like clockwork and had never misplaced or lost it. I went to the bathroom to grab another patch (my kids say there are times I should wear two or three!) and climbed back in bed. Imagine my horror when my husband got up to shower and my patch was stuck on his back! Needless to say, he had a shower partner that day and seemed to enjoy having his back lathered up! It still cracks me up to think that he might have walked around all day with female hormones coursing through his veins!

let their looks get in the way, but they do sometimes let their wife's appearance become a stumbling block. With the pervasiveness of fashion magazines, swimsuit models, television "beauties," and Internet pornography, many men are getting tainted by the cultural message regarding female beauty. If your husband is one of those men, have a truthful conversation with him about how his obsession with the world's standard of beauty is destroying his intimacy with you. If the problem persists, get professional help.

I know what it is like to have a husband who wants you to have a perfect body. I was married the first time at twenty-one to a man who would not walk down the aisle until I weighed 120 pounds. He told me how to eat and what to wear because it was important to him to have a thin wife. In *Scale Down*, I told how this obsession with my looks drove me deeper into my eating disorder and increased the damage to my already poor body image. The point is this: we have enough trouble seeing ourselves accurately; we don't need any help from the men in our lives. Yet this can be a huge problem. No matter what issues your husband has or whether he chooses to resolve them or not, *you* must learn to see yourself as a beautiful woman.

A Word for Men . . . from a Man

Throughout our marriage, my husband, Lew, has been incredibly tolerant of my female phases. He was initiated in the first few years when in my midthirties I experienced what I called my "quarterly Psycho-PMS." Many times I felt like jumping out of my skin and had zero tolerance for anything, including myself. Those days were tough, but they were simply boot camp for what was on the horizon when I began menopause. Here's what Lew has to say about it:

Have you asked yourself recently, "Who IS this person sharing my bed?" One minute she's too hot, the next too cold. What used to be great is now terrible. She used to want to be around you every waking moment and now she wants more "me time." What is going on?

Welcome to menopause, my friend! For a lucky few it will come and go with little fanfare. However, some wives will go from severe PMS in their thirties to extreme "MM" (menopause madness) in their forties and fifties.

As men (and humans), our natural inclination is one of selfishness. Our thoughts and words are often clouded in "I" or "me." "Why is she treating me this way?" "What have I done?" "I don't deserve any of this!" And you know what? You don't. Neither does she.

Danna and I had always been very close. Even in the most stressful of times, we loved being around each other and were absolutely comfortable with one another. Our goal was always to spend as much time with each other as possible.

Even after we were married for eleven years, people often mistook us for newlyweds (albeit older ones, but newlyweds just the same). But with the "change" (an appropriate moniker, don't you think?) came real changes. Danna desired more time alone. My funny little habits or nuances that used to make her laugh now annoyed her, and our very healthy level of intimacy took a severe hit.

Throughout this book, Danna provides a reasoned, God-centered approach for women to take in their journey through menopause. I love that word *journey*. It is more than just a trip. For me, living with Danna has always meant adventure, and an adventure is always best when shared. It is our decision whether our wives (the woman that God has chosen for us) take the journey alone or with the man that they married. It took me a while to understand this. It took even more time for me to gather the courage to actually talk to Danna about it. (After all, if I don't bring it up and we don't talk about it, won't it all just go away?)

Your wife may want a little more space. She may be a little edgy, moody, or downright difficult. It doesn't mean she doesn't love you or want to talk about it!

Hormone-Healthy Hints from an HHH Survivor

1. *Pray with your wife.* If you have never done this, *start*. It took me years to understand that true intimacy is not the connection that you have sexually with your wife; it is the shared intimacy you have with her through Christ.

2. *Empathize with her.* Understand that she doesn't want to go through this any more than you! But she has no choice. It is time for us as men of God to accept the meaning of the word *sacrifice*! Believe it or not, she knows that she is being an irritation to you and the entire family, whether it shows externally or not.

3. *Accept reality and change your expectations.* Accept the fact that "things" are going to be changing. The woman you married may break down occasionally. She cannot be the Proverbs 31 woman every day of her life. (I think *that* woman is a compilation of all the good qualities a woman can have rolled into one example.) Bottom line: have realistic expectations.

4. *Listen to her . . . hear her.* Ask her what connotes love to her now. It could be as simple as just listening (hint: that means active listening . . . not just hearing her talk). Maybe she needs time alone. (Hey, this is a chance for you to get to know your children better!) Or maybe she needs more help around the house. (Think of your helping hand as a good way to get a "cheap" workout, plus reacquaint yourself with the property you own or rent.)

What irritates her or makes her less than comfortable? Are your funny little nuances now irritating habits? Talk about sexual intimacy even if it is not normal for you to do so. Understand that the frequency of lovemaking may change. Never use a guilt trip to manipulate your wife into having sex. Try to understand what's going on in her mind and body. Whether her concern is emotional or physical, she may need time to adjust to the huge changes occurring.

5. *Pray with your wife.* Yes, I know I already said this. This is what I call a "reinforcement" to emphasize an important point. Prayer is the most powerful tool you have to connect both of you supernaturally to the only One who has any control over your life.

Do you remember when your dad had "the talk" with you? Boy, I sure wish dear old Dad would have clued me in to this "menopause thing." Men, take heart. Like all journeys, it is not the end that you talk about; it is the path taken and the times shared. It is up to you, with our Lord's strength, to come alongside that wonderful woman you married. And most likely you'll need to pick her up and carry her now and then. Show her the man whom God intended *you* to be.

My friend, I pray for your strength on this roller-coaster trip. I pray you'll apply God's wisdom to your specific challenges. I pray for you to be courageous, when lesser men would "cut and run." I pray blessings on you, your family, and your marriage.

Oh . . . and welcome to the HHH Club!

HEALTH FLASH

TIPS FOR HOLY HOTTIES

Sex, Sex . . . What Sex?

Hormone levels, stress, depression, low energy, and a variety of medical conditions can impact a woman's sex drive in major ways. Whether she's experiencing low libido, vaginal dryness, or pain during intercourse due to a thin vaginal wall, testing her estrogen, progesterone, testosterone, and DHEA levels can help shed light on how to best address this issue. (Of course, these tests should be done anyway if menopause symptoms persist after trying non-hormone therapies.)

Testosterone plays a key role in sexual desire for both men and women. It is imperative that women dealing with low libidos avoid taking any type of hormone without first being tested. If testosterone levels are low, replacement can be helpful in relieving vaginal dryness, maintaining bone density, increasing lean muscle mass, and possibly protecting against heart disease. Used in combination with estrogen therapy, testosterone can reduce hot flashes, night sweats, insomnia, and other symptoms that may have not sufficiently responded to estrogen alone. Too much testosterone, however, can lead to facial hair and other unwanted side effects. Use of this hormone must be closely monitored. For some women, simply balancing the progesterone/estrogen levels is enough.

According to some experts, vaginal dryness and atrophy can also be treated by local hormones for women who don't want to be on systemic therapy. Women can use a vaginal moisturizer such as Replens and a lubricant such as KY Jelly or Astroglide at the time of intercourse to deal with persistent dryness.

Committed to taking the most natural and simple route first, Dr. Mark Stengler uses herbs such as ginseng (especially Chinese or panax ginseng), puncture vine, damiana, and potency wood, which can be helpful for addressing issues related to libido and vaginal discomfort. In addition, homeopathic medicines such as sepia work well to improve libido without risk of toxicity. He also recommends trying soy foods to improve vaginal lubrication. Tofu, miso, and tempeh are good sources of soy proteins. Fermented soy powders used in shakes and smoothies may also be helpful. Vitamin E in daily doses of 800 to 1,200 IU may also help with vaginal dryness. Black cohosh may help as well; the recommended dosage is 80 to 160 milligrams.

As already discussed, libido and sexual arousal are closely connected to the mind and emotions. No hormone or supplement will ever take the place of good communication and connection with your spouse. Equally important are adequate rest, regular exercise, quality nutrition, and good stress management. When we take good care of ourselves—body, soul, and spirit—our bodies and souls respond in the most positive ways.

Taking Action

1. What was the most important truth you gained from this chapter?
2. What changes, if any, do you desire to make related to that truth?
3. What specific thoughts or actions need to be implemented to make those changes?
4. What are your greatest stumbling blocks toward this change?
5. On a scale from one to ten (with ten being the highest) how important is this relative to other needs/changes in your life? Use this scale to help you create an overall action plan when you finish reading this book.

14

Menopause and the Single Woman

Since I've spent almost thirty of my fifty-two years married, my words on singleness would have little relevance. While physically, our marital status has little impact on how menopause impacts our lives, it certainly can impact our attitudes. Sometimes the onset of menopause says to a single midlife woman, "You're too old for love." Or worse yet, some women think that they are "less than" if they spend their mature years single.

With that in mind, I sought wisdom from four unique women with somewhat different life situations. I think they all have healthy attitudes toward singleness. If you are approaching menopause and single, I hope you find their words encouraging.

Three of these women are my friends; the other is a well-known author and speaker. They all have balanced and profound things to say about singleness. They all share transparently about living as single midlife women in what some would consider a "married world."

Words of Wisdom from Diana (never married)

Have you ever placed a personal ad to meet a man? Here's one that was placed *for* me (without my permission):

Searching for a man named Russell who is tall and wears a size 12 bowling shoe. Voluptuous redhead is waiting. Call 500–1234.

Why Russell? Russell was the name engraved on the used bowling ball I received as a practical joke from a friend years ago. It also came with a bag and size 12 bowling shoes. I joked that the bowling ball was my "glass slipper," and I would try it on the fingers of every Russell I met until I found my Prince Charming (or improved my handicap, whichever came first). When my co-workers determined my quest for Russell wasn't moving quickly enough, they decided to expedite the process by placing that ad for me in a local newspaper. Not only did they place the ad, they also recorded the greeting on the private voicemail box that interested "Russells" were directed to call (I've never sounded so sexy).

Despite their best efforts, only two men named Russell responded. The first was a part-time copy editor and late-night deejay on a local radio station. He sported a goatee and a Prince Valiant haircut. The second wasn't a Russell at all, but he had responded to ten or twelve ads that day and couldn't remember which one he was calling about. Alas, the bowling ball remained in its bag.

I gained several interesting insights from my Russell experience, though:

1) My co-workers had WAY too much free time on their hands;

2) I will never marry a man with a Prince Valiant haircut;
3) The key to "successful singleness" is perspective.[1]

Get out of the Waiting Room

Most women think of singleness as "doing time until I get married." We live in a kind of "holding pattern" until we find a mate. We wait for Mr. Right like we would wait for a doctor's appointment—sitting in the waiting room, distracting ourselves with whatever's available, waiting for someone to call our name. Our focus is on how we got here, and our perspective becomes limited to our condition and what it will take to "get over it." Singleness is not a sickness. It's not something we have to "get over." I've learned that my purpose in life is in the here and now, not in the somewhere and someday. It's important to plan and to dream, but it's even more important to live and experience.

Jump in the Water

I recently went to Hawaii with a couple of girlfriends. One of the issues I had to deal with was "The Bathing Suit." I don't look good in one and am rather self-conscious. I knew I couldn't compete with the bikini-clad women I anticipated would be lying around the pool. But I remember thinking to myself, *You're going to Hawaii, and a large part of the fun involves a bathing suit. Are you going to sit on the sidelines feeling sorry for yourself or are you going to jump in the water?* I decided to jump in the water.

I'm pleased to say that no one shrieked in horror when they saw me in my bathing suit. No one pointed and stared and compared my measurements to the girls in the bikinis or made me feel inadequate. The truth is, most of us were too busy having fun in the water to pay much attention to each other's appearance. Our focus was on the experience, not the impression we were making or how we measured up.

So often, we singles sit on the sidelines rather than jump in the water. Instead of being intimidated by bikinis, we're intimidated by couples. I confess I have avoided more than one company Christmas party because I didn't have a date. The same goes for weddings or other date-oriented functions. That changed when I saw a dear girlfriend of mine at a party . . . with another girlfriend. They were having a blast. I didn't think, *Oh, how sad that Susie had to bring a girlfriend instead of a "real date."* I thought, *Hey, I wish I would have thought of that. They're having a great time!* I have since attended with a "friend date" several functions that I might otherwise have skipped. I've even attended a company Christmas party alone. In every case, once I got to the event, my focus was on having fun and making new friends, not on the fact that I wasn't with my dream date.

Go ahead and jump in the water! It may be a little uncomfortable at first, but after a few minutes, it feels great! Successful singleness means living in the here and now . . . and not worrying about whether you'll have a date for it.

Find Contentment

In a letter to the Philippians, the ever-so-single apostle Paul wrote, "I have learned to be content whatever the circumstances. I know what it is to be in need, and I know what it is to have plenty. I have learned the secret of being content in any and every situation, whether well fed or hungry, whether living in plenty or in want. I can do everything through him who gives me strength. Yet it was good of you to share in my troubles" (4:11–14 NIV). I wonder if Paul's friends ever asked him about his singleness.

"Paul, you're such a wonderful man. How is it you've never been married?"

"Are you dating someone right now? No? Why not?"

"Where are you meeting people? You've gotta get out there, Paul!"

I had dinner with a married girlfriend a few years ago. She brought up the issue of my singleness and asked me who I was dating. I told her I wasn't really dating anyone at that time, and then she asked me why. I told her I didn't know. She decided to analyze the situation. "Are you afraid of commitment or of getting hurt?" "Do you have some issues with your father?" It was incomprehensible to her that I wasn't dating because I just wasn't dating. Even more amazing to her was that I was comfortable with it. Since she was a leader in our church, I mentioned Paul's words to her. "Didn't the apostle Paul say he had learned to be content in all circumstances? Well, I'm content with my circumstances, and I'm trusting God for a husband if it's in his will and timing. Isn't that a good place to be?" She sputtered for a moment and then answered, "Yeah, I guess it is."

I've noticed that a lot of the married people I know are uncomfortable with my singleness. I think they're afraid I might be lonely. Comedian Mark Lowry shares a great story about going to dinner with some married friends. They too were concerned with his singleness and one of them asked him, "Don't you ever get lonely?" He responded, "Sure, don't you?" The table then got very quiet.

Of course single people get lonely. But so do married people. Just as marriage isn't an automatic cure for loneliness, so singleness isn't an automatic sentence of loneliness. When people ask me about my singleness, I no longer get defensive and feel like I have to explain myself. The truth is, I don't know why I'm still single. I just haven't met the right man and perhaps I never will. They may not be satisfied with that answer, but it's the only one I've got. Besides, trying to explain to people why I'm single is a waste of time.

Being content in all circumstances, including singleness, is something we have to learn, and it's something that involves God. But learning to be content doesn't mean stuffing our true feelings and putting on a happy face. That's called denial. In the process of learning to be content, we need to be honest with God about our struggles and desires. Being honest doesn't mean getting on our knees and crying, "Why am I still single, God? Why haven't you sent me a mate? Why do I have to watch my friends get married while I have no one? Why? Why? Why?" That's not praying; it's whining.

Put God First

Honesty with God involves sharing our hurts and hopes: "Lord, I'm struggling with my singleness. I'm hurting and I'm lonely. Help me. Your Word says that I can do all things through Christ who strengthens me. Lord, strengthen me to be content in the place that you have me. You know that I desire to be married. It's hard to be single, Lord, but I trust you."

Being content in your singleness does not mean you have no desire for a husband. The desire to love and be loved is natural. God *created* us for relationship—with himself and with others. In the past, I got my relationships "out of order" and found myself "falling back" on my relationship with God when my relationship with someone else didn't work out. In other words, I would "settle" for spending time with God on a Friday night if there was no one asking me out. Others first, God second—what a shallow understanding I had of God!

A friend once asked me what trait I most desired in my future husband. I thought about it for a few moments and replied, "He has to 'get' me. He has to understand my deepest hopes and fears. He has to know what makes me tick, and he has to take me seriously." I shake my head when I think that I used to put God, the only One who truly "gets" me because he's the one who *created* me, in the "fallback" position of my love life.

God knows us better than we know ourselves. He knows our heart's desire to love and be loved. His words to Isaiah concerning Israel are true for us as well: "Your Maker is your husband—the LORD Almighty is his name—the Holy One of Israel is your Redeemer; he is called the God of all the earth" (Isa. 54:5 NIV).

When I have my relationships "in order"—God first, others second—my singleness isn't a big issue. God designed me to be complete in him. Whether I'm married or single, I'll only find true contentment there. Successful singleness means understanding a relationship with God is the key to every other relationship in life.

A husband isn't a substitute for God; nor is God a substitute for a husband. God *is* my husband—my relationship with him comes first. Then, when the time is right, I hope he will also bless me with a husband "with skin on." The relationship with the man I hope to marry will be in addition to, not in place of, my relationship with my Maker. I pray with the psalmist: "Teach me your way, O LORD, and I will walk in your truth; give me an undivided heart, that I may fear your name" (Ps. 86:11 NIV).

I don't have to divide my love between my earthly husband and my heavenly one. My relationship with God will multiply my ability to love others, including the man I may marry. The psalmist puts it this way: "Teach me your ways, O LORD, that I may live according to your truth! Grant me purity of heart, that I may honor you" (Ps. 86:11 NLT). A heart that is pure and devoted to him is what God seeks. What husband wouldn't want that also?

Final Thoughts

Stop asking God why you're single. Not because he doesn't know or is withholding the answer but because we tend to obsess on this kind of question and take on a "victim" mentality. Singleness is not a punishment, nor is it a defect or handicap. Being single is simply where God has you right now. Be honest with him and trust him—he loves you more than you realize and knows exactly what's best for you right now.

Don't have all the answers to the mystery of your love life? Join the club and get on with your life! Being single is tough sometimes, but so is being married. Don't focus on what's *not* happening in your life; focus on what *is*. God doesn't want you to kill time waiting for a husband; he wants you to cherish the life he's given you.

Although I continue to grow in my singleness (living in the here and now; being honest in my struggles but content in my situation; understanding that my relationship with God is what's most important), I still wonder where my "Russell" might be. I wonder if he's wondering about me. Lord, I pray you're preparing him for me as you're preparing me for him, and that he's growing closer to you every day. And most important, Lord, I pray he doesn't have a Prince Valiant haircut.

(Diana wrote this piece about six years ago . . . today she is still a contented single.)

Words of Wisdom from Terri (divorced and remarried)

Sex, love, identity, significance—these were all interrelated for me. Like anyone else, I wanted to feel special, loved, and significant. My problem in the past was that I looked for it in all the wrong places. When I reflect on my life and the choices

I have made, I see that I experienced a lot of heartbreak and shame by not following God's plan. My choices led to teenage sex and promiscuity, early marriage and divorce, a second marriage and a second divorce. My choices also led me to question the core of my identity. I always thought I was a "good" person. How could I end up with two failed marriages before I hit forty?

Life for me was like that old song sung by Dean Martin: "You're nobody 'til somebody loves you." From a very young age, girls are led to believe that when they find that "special someone," life will be perfect. They'll finally be somebody. When you buy into the myth that you're nobody 'til somebody loves you, you miss a lot of living, make decisions for the wrong reasons, and suffer the heartbreaks that follow.

Whether we label it self-esteem or self-worth, we must have a sense of significance based on truth. Understanding this emotional need will give us great insight into our actions and attitudes. As I sought to understand this need on a personal level, I had to specifically address the role men played in how I saw myself. As little girls, our first relationship with a man is the one we have with our dads. The quality of that relationship has profound influence. Mine was a bit troubled, and all my relationships with men had been troubled. So after another painful breakup—and fearing yet another failure—I decided to seek Christian counseling and begin a healing process.

My therapist told me not to enter another relationship for six months. At that time, I wasn't sure I could last that long. I'd been dependent on men for my identity since I was fifteen years old. But I decided to give it a go. I went on what I refer to as my "Man Fast," and it lasted over two years. It turned out to be a great season in my life—a tremendous period of growth. In the process, I began to see my singleness as a gift.

I realized that I needed to be healed inside before I could ever make choices that would lead me to a healthy relationship. My assignment was to establish my own identity, apart from any man or any other person in my life for that matter. I needed to be *whole*. If I could be whole, I could enter a relationship without needing someone to complete me or make me feel significant. If *I* could be whole, I could attract a *whole* man. Think of people waiting for a bone transplant. They need to find someone who is suitable. Their problem isn't that no one cares or is willing to share their gift of life, but it is essential a right match be found. The body won't bond with something that is unfamiliar and neither should you.

Today, I am married to a wonderful match. But I can honestly say that my years of "man fasting" were some of the best of my life. If the right mate had not come along, I truly believe I could have been content being single for much longer.

(For those of you who feel your biological clock is ticking, Terri just had her first [and she says only] child at forty-one years old. We kid that she is "one and done at forty-one!")

Words of Wisdom from Sandi (divorced)

My friend Sandi found herself in a different life situation at fifty. After thirty years of marriage to one man, she was suddenly single under very difficult circumstances. I interviewed Sandi about her unique experiences and perspectives. This is what she shared.

Q: What are the hardest things about being single and menopausal?

A: There is a sense of loss of femininity with the changes. It is hard to see and feel the changes in your body and not have anyone around to affirm you. I was going through a divorce and menopause at the same time. Insecurity abounded in me. With sleeplessness as one of my symptoms, I found the nights long and very lonely.

Q: What are the best things about being single and menopausal?

A: Sleeping nude when the hot flashes hit and not worrying if I look fat! Realizing this is not a "hidden disease." Taking comfort in the fact that there is much humor and support out there in books like this one, movies like *The First Wives Club*, and so forth. Thankfully, it's much different from when our mothers went through it.

Q: How does God fill in the gaps for a single woman?

A: God has led me gently through hard times and decisions that I have had to make. He has never made me search for him; he has laid my path clearly out for me. My intimacy with God through my single time made me realize that intimacy with a man could never be as intense or constant as my intimacy with him. His closeness to me in my times of tears and prayer and his gently leading me have made me realize I would never want to lose it by simply transferring that to a man. Rather, I would bring all God has given me into a husband/wife relationship (if that were to happen) with another believer, making our marriage so much richer.

Q: How do girlfriends fill in the gaps?

A: We laugh, cry, complain, pray, eat, work out, and so forth. We have challenged one another to revel in our femininity. Pink sheets with polka dots might be a bit much for a husband but are great for a single. My single girlfriends and I have learned to vacation together, try new and sometimes daring things, push our bodies to the max, keep one another accountable, and gently lift one another when we are in the dumps. In fact, sometimes we just sit in the dumps together with a box of chocolates, Starbucks, and a warm blanket.

Q: Do you enjoy single more than married girlfriends? Why?

A: No, I don't. After having been engaged/married for over thirty years, I enjoy the company of a man. My friends' husbands are very important to me. I have recently lost my brother and father and feel God has given me these "safe" men to enjoy. They will be my dance partners, tell me I look nice, tease me, offer to fix what is broken in my apartment, and sometimes give me the kind of hug only a man can give. That feels nice!

Q: What is the best tip you have for dealing with menopause madness?

A: Remember, this (like being thirteen to fifteen years old!!) is only a "season." If we fight it, deny it, hate it, or become embittered because of it, we will miss what God would have us learn in this stage. It isn't forever (though some nights it feels like it is). Be educated; keep moving; listen to your unique body; learn the best way to care for yourself; and don't forget to laugh!

A Few Words from Danna

Okay, I know I said I had nothing to say about being single, but I do have something to say about being rejected. Most of us go through rejection in one form or another in our lives. It often leaves us single for a very painful season. I was rejected a couple times in my life: by my first true love at eighteen and later when my husband was unfaithful for a short time.

Both were agonizing times for me. How do you deal with rejection? Is a past hurt stopping you from even exploring relationships today? I love the little verse that encourages us to live life to the fullest without excuses. It says:

> Work like you don't need the money.
> Love like you've never been hurt.
> Dance like no one is watching.

Rejected Again?

If you are in the midst of menopause, not only single, but single because the man in your life has rejected you, my heart goes out to you. It takes time, truth, and authentic connection with One who fully loves you to heal a broken heart.

Watching the reality show *The Bachelor* gave me an insight into how our perspective impacts our response to rejection. On the show, an attractive young bachelor was presented with a challenge to find the "perfect wife" from among twenty or more women who had been selected based on criteria he'd provided. Over the course of many episodes, he would eliminate candidates until he had chosen only one who would potentially become his wife.

As the show progressed, he reduced his choice to the top five candidates. At the end of each episode, he would present a single red rose to those he wanted to pursue and "reject" just one. Something in me wanted to scream, "This isn't fair! Why would these women subject themselves to this kind of potential rejection?" In the end, with two candidates remaining, the bachelor struggled with his decision and seemed genuinely concerned about choosing the "right one." He presented his single red rose to his chosen one, and a rejected young lady rode off alone in a limousine.

Chosen by God

If we pursue intimate relationships, we risk rejection—that is, if the relationship is with another human. God, however, is incapable of rejecting you. If you know him yet don't "feel" loved and chosen, it is time you fully embrace the profound and limitless love he has to pour out on you, his beloved. Every time you ask, he responds enthusiastically with, "I choose you!" And he confirms his love, not with a single red rose but with something far more precious, far more costly—his Son's blood.

I learned in my times of deep despair that God alone can fill the gaps in our hearts left oozing with bitterness and fear from rejection. His love is perfect, complete, and eternal. But we must believe and we must receive this profound truth for ourselves. If we marry the man of our dreams but never spend time with him or share our deepest thoughts, we would still feel alone. That goes for our relationship with God as well. If we draw close to God through Christ, he will draw close to us. And while his love doesn't ensure that we will never be hurt by the "less than perfect" who roam this fallen world, it will sustain us and give us courage to risk again.

It is natural after experiencing rejection and betrayal to blame another person. We may even blame God; after all, he allowed it to happen, didn't he? Unfortunately, until we reach heaven, we will experience pain in this fallen world. In the meantime we must remember that God will never reject us. Once we are his, he will pursue us with a passion. And he does . . . even if we don't feel it.

Whether the holes in your heart are due to betrayal, neglect, or simply a poor concept of who you really are in Christ, you need restoration. God loves all who believe in the name of his Son. Without that truth penetrating you to the very core, you will seek significance and satisfaction in all the wrong places.

Luci Swindoll—Single by Choice

While I was struggling with exactly how to approach this chapter on singleness, I just "happened" to catch a Focus on the Family radio program. It was a replay of an interview Dr. James Dobson had done with popular author, speaker, and Women of Faith team member Luci Swindoll; the subject was singleness.

Many years ago Luci wrote a book called *Wide My World . . . Narrow My Bed*. She shared that, at age ten, she realized she wanted to remain single throughout her life. Luci seemed to know that she had a lot of adventure in her and wanted the freedom to travel and explore life without the pressure of a husband or children. Another of her books, *I Married Adventure*, is filled with color photos she has taken in her world travels.

Luci says she sees every aspect of life as an adventure. However, when she began speaking to singles groups, she noticed tremendous disappointment, anger, and even bitterness among many older singles. She thinks singles can live fully by looking at the possibilities of today rather than wishing for the uncertain hopes for tomorrow.

Luci addresses the issue of life's disappointments, stating, "When a spouse walks out or dies or a child turns against you or you're 50 and still single, life is going to be only what you make it. If you don't look at it from that point of view, you will experience tremendous disappointment, because you expect something that is not under your control."

Dr. Dobson shared an important insight from a man's perspective. He said, "If we continue to pine for something we do not have, we are not very attractive to other people. You need to do the things you want to do whether you are married or single."

In the closing moments of the interview, Dr. Dobson read these words from the last page of Luci's book. In it she writes:

> My dear single friend, if I could close this book with one ringing message in your ears, it would be to once again encourage you to get into the enthusiasm of living. Don't wait for a mate. Don't wait for time. Don't wait until you have more money. Don't wait until you get both feet back on the ground. Don't wait for anything else. The time to be involved with living is now—not tomorrow or next week—but now![2]

HEALTH FLASH
TIPS FOR HOLY HOTTIES

Healthy Recipes for Holy Hotties

Single or married, we all have to eat. I've included some favorite recipes that are nutritious and taste great. Get creative and find ways to add nutrient-dense foods to your meals and recipes. For example, chop up kale and other veggies and add them to your spaghetti sauces, stews, and soups. Use olive oil when cooking or making salads and slip a little tofu into a recipe now and then. Get creative and eat for life!

PEANUTTY ENERGY BARS
Mix together in a medium bowl and set aside:
½ cup salted dry-roasted peanuts
½ cup roasted shelled sunflower seeds
¼ cup toasted wheat germ
½ cup raisins or dried cranberries

2 cups uncooked oatmeal (not instant)
2 cups toasted rice cereal
¼ cup flaxseed

Combine the following in a large bowl and microwave on high for 2 minutes:
½ cup crunchy peanut butter
½ cup firmly packed brown sugar
½ cup light corn syrup

Add a teaspoon of vanilla and stir until blended. Add dry ingredients gradually and stir until coated. Spoon mixture into an 8-inch square pan coated with nonstick cooking spray. Press down firmly (it helps to spray fingers with nonstick spray). Let stand about 1 hour and cut into bars. Makes 16 servings. Each serving: 260 calories, 13.8 grams fat, 5.82 grams protein, 32 grams carbohydrates.

SALMON WITH MAPLE SYRUP AND TOASTED ALMONDS

Six 6-ounce salmon fillets
Cooking spray
¼ cup packed brown sugar
¼ cup maple syrup
3 tablespoons low-sodium soy sauce
1 tablespoon Dijon mustard
¼ teaspoon black pepper
4 teaspoons sliced almonds, toasted

Preheat oven to 425° F. Place fillets in a 13 x 9-inch baking dish coated with cooking spray. Combine sugar, syrup, soy sauce, mustard, and black pepper; pour sugar mixture over fillets. Cover with foil; bake at 425° for 10 minutes. Remove foil; sprinkle the fillets with almonds. Bake an additional 10 minutes or until fish flakes easily when tested with a fork. Serve with sugar mixture. Yields 6 servings. Each serving: 373 calories, 12.78 grams fat, 43.42 grams protein, 19 grams carbohydrates.

POTATO AND BELL PEPPER FRITTATA

1 tablespoon olive oil
8 ounces red-skinned potatoes, thinly sliced
½ cup sliced red onion
½ of a red bell pepper, thinly sliced

½ of a yellow bell pepper, thinly sliced
½ cup broccoli, chopped
2 teaspoons fresh chopped sage or dried rubbed sage
1 teaspoon salt
½ teaspoon freshly ground pepper
8 eggs
2¼ cups finely shredded Parmesan cheese

1. Preheat oven to 350° F. Heat olive oil in a 12-inch nonstick ovenproof skillet over medium heat. Add potatoes, onion, bell peppers, and broccoli; cover and cook, stirring occasionally, until vegetables are tender, 10 minutes. Stir in 1 teaspoon of the sage, ½ teaspoon of the salt, and ¼ teaspoon of the pepper.

2. Whisk together the eggs, 2 cups of the cheese, and the remaining sage, salt, and pepper; pour over vegetables in skillet and cook until edges of eggs just begin to set, 3 minutes.

3. Sprinkle top with the remaining cheese and bake until center is set, 8 minutes. Invert onto a serving plate. Makes 4 servings. Each serving: 435 calories, 27 grams fat, 33 grams protein, 14 grams carbohydrates.

BOK CHOY SALAD WITH CRUNCHIES
1 bunch bok choy
1 bunch green onions
1 head green or purple cabbage

Salad Dressing
¾ cup oil
⅓ cup sugar
¼ cup wine vinegar
2 tablespoons soy sauce

Crunchies
2 packages crumbled ramen noodles
½ cup sesame seeds
1¾ cup sliced almonds

Sauté crunchies until brown in ½ cup butter and 2 tablespoons sugar. Stir constantly. Lay out on paper towels to cool. Makes enough crunchy toppings for two salads. Makes 10 servings. Each serving: 349 calories, 30.81 grams fat, 4.86 grams protein, 17 grams carbohydrates.

Taking Action

1. What was the most important truth you gained from this chapter?
2. What changes, if any, do you desire to make related to that truth?
3. What specific thoughts or actions need to be implemented to make those changes?
4. What are your greatest stumbling blocks toward this change?
5. On a scale from one to ten (with ten being the highest) how important is this relative to other needs/changes in your life? Use this scale to help you create an overall action plan when you finish reading this book.

15

You Can't Take It with You

How do you measure your success in life thus far? If you use the world's standards you might buy into the bumper-sticker philosophy that exclaims: "He who dies with the most toys wins!" (My pastor says, "He who dies with the most toys . . . is dead!") As we get older, we sometimes give in to the false notion that we should have made more money, had a better home, and secured better things to pass on to our kids. At some level, we believe that a big part of our legacy will be our worldly possessions.

By the time we hit menopause, we've accumulated tons of stuff. In fact, if we didn't have so much, we probably wouldn't need so many rooms in our houses.

One of my favorite mentors, Florence Littauer, says we need to learn the difference between need and greed. Once our primary needs for food, clothing, and shelter are satisfied,

---

Ode to My "Stuff"

I'm turning fifty-two and I'm packing too much stuff.
My purse is overloaded, yet it never holds enough.

Shoes are in abundance and my closet overflows.
But, when there's some place to go, I can't find the right clothes.

Lipstick tubes, mascara, and eye shadows galore;
Then, I discover a new product and get "just one more."

What never gets too full to take on added cargo
Are those ever-expanding fat cells turning me into a "lardo."

Days are long and life gets hard, the challenges are whopping,
When stress is high, I seek relief . . . I eat or do some shopping!

Travel light, my friend, as you approach your final destination.
The stuff you've got is all but naught when you reach your
   jubilation!

So, let it go. Give it away. Gather things that matter.
Hugs and kisses; smiles and laughs . . . these things will never
   shatter.

And when your final day has come and to the dust you do return;
Just leave your "tent" with all your stuff—take the prize you never
   earned.

He's waiting with a mansion, a glorious body to one day behold.
The stuff you had is worthless; his rewards are precious gold.

---

we don't really "need" all that much. I try to remember that when I peruse the fashion catalogs that come in the mail or insist that I "need" a pair of sage green shoes to match my sage green suit.

Don't get me wrong. I'm not planning to give everything away tomorrow and become like Mother Teresa. But I do have a personal need to know that if I must let go of it earlier than expected, I can do so with grace.

Fiery Trials

In the past, I've been inspired and humbled by stories of people who have lost all their worldly possessions. I've tried to imagine what it would be like to have only the clothes on my back. Recently, I came pretty close to losing everything. I wrote much of this chapter in the midst of that fiery trial.

Sunday, October 26, 2003, 3:00 p.m.

The heat is on in San Diego, but it's not because we're having a huge convention of menopausal women. In all seriousness, as I write these words, wildfires, flamed by erratic Santa Ana winds, have taken Southern California and especially our county by storm. This afternoon ten lives have been lost and at least a hundred homes consumed. Since early morning, the sky has been dark and ash has been falling, remnants of once green trees or someone's personal belongings. I brushed grayish white residue off my shoulders as I entered church this morning, wondering from what source it had originated. An eerie, surrealistic glow has enveloped us. The sun is bright red behind the dark haze. I've never been one to worry unduly, but I'm a bit worried right now. It's the first day back on standard time and sunset is arriving early. The wind and fire show no sign of slowing down.

Sunday, 11:00 p.m.

Things have changed a bit since I wrote my last words. We've packed our cars with as many important belongings as they will hold and left our home not sure if we'll see it again. After the police came through our neighborhood with bullhorns telling us we should consider evacuating, I took a walk through each room. You can accumulate a lot living twelve years in one place. It amazed me how little I really cared about all those objects. I don't want to lose them. It would be inconvenient to start over. But if we have to, I know it will happen because God allows it. We're praying he will protect our home, but our major concern is that he protects *us*.

We weren't in a huge hurry to get out tonight. There was no sense of panic, just concern. It was odd trying to decide what to take. Of course, pictures cannot be replaced. Important files or tax documents seemed worth packing. My laptop computer was on the top of my list—this book was in the hard drive!

Jesse had different priorities. I put a big green bin in the middle of his room and told him he could fill it with what he wanted to take. I bit my tongue when I saw it full of action figures and cars and fought my inclination to make suggestions. We put it in the SUV with all his "treasures"; he had a small sense of control in an uncontrollable situation.

Now we sit watching the local news at my friend's house a few miles away. More than six hundred homes have been destroyed so far today in Southern California. Thirteen people are reported dead. We prayed as a group before we brushed our teeth and attempted to grab a few hours' sleep on the couch. It's hard to know how to pray. I keep remembering how Jesus calmed the storm on the lake when the disciples were terrified. We're scared too. We prayed for the winds to still so we could hear critical breaking information on television. Flames are licking the hills to our east and south. These two fires of unique origins are like allied forces trying to capture us from two fronts. We slept fitfully, wondering how many homes and lives would be lost before dawn.

Monday Morning

Our home is still standing; our neighborhood hasn't been touched! A half inch of ash has dusted everything, but who cares? Every school in the county is closed, and almost everyone is staying home from work. For the moment our homes look safe. But all over the county the damage has increased overnight and more people have lost absolutely every earthly possession. Most folks interviewed on radio and television have the right perspective . . . they are thankful to be alive. They know their losses are only "stuff." It's hard; it's inconvenient; but it's temporal.

In the midst of all the chaos of the last day, my friend Jeff had to deal with a more significant loss. After receiving the command to evacuate their neighborhood, he and his family got a call on their cell phone as their overpacked car headed out. His mom had just died. Yet even in the middle of that devastating news, there was reason to celebrate. Jeff's mother, Marie, had cried out in excruciating pain and begged God to take her home. The cancer diagnosed only weeks ago was ravaging her body faster than the wildfires were burning San Diego. She knew the Lord, and he delivered her mercifully from prolonged anguish. He is a God of love and compassion. We must remember that in the most trying of times.

Treasures in Heaven

Time after time, I've heard Christians dealing with life's heartaches quote Romans 8:28: "And we know that God causes all things to work together for good to those who love God, to those who are called according to His purpose." When we read the verse in context, we find that the "good" is realized in eternity, not on earth. In Romans 8:18 Paul writes, "For I consider that the sufferings of this present time are not worthy to be compared with the glory that is to be revealed to us." He goes on to summarize the "sufferings" we endure on this fallen planet in verse 22: "For we know that the whole creation groans and suffers the pains of childbirth together until now."

Paul then speaks of the hope we stand in during our trials in verse 25: "But if we hope for what we do not see, with perseverance we wait eagerly for it." What is the hope? Is it finding a way out of today's difficulties? No. It is the hope of our salvation—knowing that all the blessings God has stored up for us will be realized in heaven.

The week of the fires, my radio partner and I discussed on our daily show the devastation from the fires that scorched much of Southern California. We heard many accounts of people who were spared. Several recounted that all the homes in their neighborhood were burned to cinders with one exception—theirs. Our callers were praising God for answering their prayers and sparing them and their "stuff."

Yes, God is to be praised, but I couldn't help thinking that in the bigger picture those who lost all their worldly possessions would ultimately be the most "blessed." Most of us don't have the inclination (or courage) to let go of everything, especially later in life when we have worked so hard to have a nice home and some financial security. I am increasingly convinced, though, that I must learn to hold my stuff as if it were sand slipping through my fingers.

I am reminded of a comment a man from a Third World country made while visiting America. When asked how he liked our country, he answered, "It is a wonderful place; full of many blessings. It seems that most people do not have to worry about having enough food to eat or adequate shelter.

Their worries are about their cars running properly or if they can pay off all their credit card bills. I am anxious to get home where each and every day I must depend upon Jesus to meet my most basic needs. I fear if I lived in America, I would forget how much I need Jesus."

Temporal Blessings

Most of the promises God gives us in his Word with respect to this temporal life are pretty basic. Look at what Jesus said about the worries of meeting our physical needs in Matthew 6:25: "For this reason I say to you, do not be worried about your life, as to what you will eat or what you will drink; nor for your body, as to what you will put on. Is not life more than food, and the body more than clothing?" He goes on to say in verses 32–34: "For your heavenly Father knows that you need all these things. But seek first His kingdom and His righteousness, and all these things will be added to you. So do not worry about tomorrow; for tomorrow will care for itself. Each day has enough trouble of its own."

That's great advice. If Jesus said it, it should be possible to let go of the worry about the "stuff" we need, shouldn't it? But some things are hard to let go of and some days are worse than others. We must always try to understand biblical truth and let that truth penetrate not only our minds but our very souls. When knowledge becomes personal belief, our emotions will follow. And when the Holy Spirit animates the Word of God in our lives, we walk not by the flesh but by the Spirit.

If we have a false notion that temporal "blessings" are God's reward for living well or a report card for our spirituality, we are sadly mistaken. Look at the life of Paul. Here was a man called by direct revelation from Christ Jesus himself, but he had more trials and tribulations than most of us could ever hope to endure. However, from his thorn in the flesh, to shipwrecks, jailing, and condemnation, Paul's total focus was Christ.

We can learn a lot about dealing with life from Paul. He writes from his jail cell in Philippians 4:4: "Rejoice in the Lord always; again I will say, rejoice!" Two verses later, he tells us to "be anxious for nothing, but in everything by prayer and supplication with thanksgiving let your requests be made known to God" (v. 6). Then, no matter what the result, the promise in verse 7 is: "And the peace of God, which surpasses all comprehension, will guard your hearts and your minds in Christ Jesus."

Think about what it means to have the peace of God guard your heart and mind. To me, it means I will be so enthralled with the love of God and his ultimate purpose for me that I will endure with joy and perseverance whatever blessings or losses life delivers.

My husband and I have been blessed in recent years with more material wealth than we expected. We're not rich by any means, but life is comfortable, and we are able to live and give beyond our expectations.

I used to think that if we simply tithed and were generous with our material wealth, God was somehow obligated to give back to us, "pressed down, shaken together, and running over" (Luke 6:38). I didn't realize until my pastor took me back to the full context of that verse that it has nothing to do with material blessing. The objects of the pressing, shaking, and running over are mercy and judgment. Read verses 36 and 37; it's pretty clear. My point is that whenever our motive is "getting," God rarely responds with "giving."

This is not to say that we cannot accumulate wealth and material things simply by working hard. We can. And, we often do (in the flesh). I heard Mel Gibson say in an interview recently that despite the fact that he had "achieved it all—the money and the fame" he was still empty until he sought the Lord. We may not know why God allows some to prosper with moderate "sweat" and others to beat their brows for a lifetime and assess very little in the material realm. Yet in the eternal perspective we will see who truly was the most "blessed."

A couple years ago, my husband and I bought a luxury car. We decided on one that was two years old and saved a lot of money. Nevertheless, I felt both guilty and conspicuous at times, thinking perhaps we were being too materialistic. One day, my twenty-two-year-old daughter, Jill, was riding with me and asked, "Mom, what's it like having everything you want?"

Whoa! That question caught me off guard for a moment. Then, with a quick prayer and the gift of God's wisdom, I answered, "I'm not sure, Jill. The things that really matter to me, I cannot buy. I couldn't buy you out of a pregnancy at fifteen years old or your sister out of prison for trafficking drugs. I couldn't buy myself out of sixteen years of bulimia or five years of overwhelming panic attacks. I can't buy my friends out of cancer or my heart out of breaking when someone rejects me. These things that I have are simply that—things. They sometimes make life easier and for a moment slightly more enjoyable, but they leave little lasting satisfaction."

I read a story about a wealthy man who, like me, wanted his child to see life accurately. He took his son on a trip to the country to visit an underprivileged family with the firm purpose of showing him how poor people can be. They spent a whole day and night on the simple farm.

When they got back from the trip the father asked his son, "So, how did you like the trip?"

"Very well, Dad!"

"Did you see how poor people can be?" the father asked.

"Yeah!"

"And what did you learn, Son?"

The son answered, "I saw that we have a dog at home, and they have four. We have a pool that reaches to the middle of the garden; they have a creek that has no end. We have imported lamps in the yard; they have the stars. Our patio reaches to the end of our property; they have the whole horizon."

When the boy was finished, the father was speechless. His son added, "Thanks, Dad, for showing me how poor we are!"

Sometimes, we need a paradigm shift to celebrate the blessings that are right under our noses. We look at what the world has to offer and in our humanness covet all that is tantalizing our desires. When you look at the wonders of the world, what do you behold as great?

A group of students were asked to list what they thought were the present "Seven Wonders of the World." After collecting their papers, the teacher listed on the chalkboard those that received the most votes. The winners were:

1. Egypt's Great Pyramids
2. Taj Mahal
3. Grand Canyon
4. Panama Canal
5. Empire State Building
6. St. Peter's Basilica
7. China's Great Wall

At the end of the exercise, the teacher noticed that one student had not finished his paper. She asked him why and the young boy replied, "I couldn't make up my mind because there were so many." Thinking he might have an interesting consideration for their list, she answered, "Well, tell us what you have and maybe we can help." The boy hesitated and then read his "Seven Wonders of the World":

1. To see
2. To hear
3. To touch
4. To taste
5. To feel
6. To laugh
7. And to love

I'm sure the room was so quiet you could have heard a pin drop. It is easy to take for granted the most wondrous blessings and possessions. We need this kind of reminder in the firestorms of life.

If you celebrate with gratitude all God has given you for today, you will be truly blessed. In this season of life, I think there are a few important principles we need to embrace and pass on.

1. You can't take it with you.
2. What you have isn't yours.
3. Give, give, and give some more as unto the Lord.
4. Don't measure your worth by material wealth.

In Matthew 6:20–21 Jesus says, "But store up for yourselves treasures in heaven, where neither moth nor rust destroys, and where thieves do not break in or steal; for where your treasure is, there your heart will be also." All of our security and joy in this life on earth and in heaven depends upon believing and living out this truth.

Every day, I must ask myself in the midst of living, *Where is your heart, Danna?* Without "setting my mind on things above" it seems to always want to default to the "human setting" that screams "I need!" "I want!" "I must have!" When life heats up for you (beyond the flashes) and you fear loss of any kind, ask yourself this question: What is the absolute worst thing that could happen?

Whether the loss involves material things, emotional security, or even a cherished loved one, there is only one permanent and devastating loss to truly fear. That would be for you or someone you know to die without knowing Christ. If you know him but fear for another . . . share the good news and pray diligently for that person. It is not your job to save him or her. It is God's. But for some miraculous reason, he has included us in the wondrous blessing of being part of his plan to draw fallen people to himself.

On a personal level, the only thing that got me through the years that my daughters were in outrageous rebellion was the fact that despite their behavior they had a saving faith in Christ. They certainly weren't living it out. But I knew they knew him as Savior.

If you do not have a personal relationship with Jesus Christ, please carefully consider the following paragraphs with an open heart and mind.

God loves you and wants to have a relationship with you—a personal, intimate, life-changing relationship. If you are not absolutely positive that you know God intimately through the sacrifice of his Son, Jesus Christ, then I challenge you to ask yourself what you believe. If you were to die today and stand before God and he were to ask you, "Why should I let you in to my heaven?" what would you say?

The familiar verse John 3:16 tells us how to receive eternal life: "For God so loved the world, that He gave His only begotten Son, that whoever believes in Him shall not perish, but have eternal life." It's that simple. Believe in the Son. Later in the same book of John, chapter 14, verse 6, Jesus said, "I am the way, and the truth, and the life; no one comes to the Father but through Me." God never refuses to save anyone who believes. Yet he does not force anyone to accept.

Once we truly understand that God's holiness and our imperfection are incompatible, we begin to appreciate why Christ came and died. In Romans 3:23, the Bible says, "All have sinned and fall short of the glory of God." That means everyone. And the most common sin of all is self-sufficiency. We don't think we need God. He also says in Romans 6:23 that "the wages of sin is death." (That is eternal separation from God, a.k.a. hell.)

The rules governing who goes to heaven or hell are established by God's nature and are unchangeable. He is the judge and jury. A perfect sacrifice for sin is required. That sacrifice is Christ. If you accept Christ's death as the payment for your sin—past, present, and future—you are cleansed and made holy. Christ not only died but rose from the dead to new life. When you believe, you experience a spiritual birth and are reborn as a child of God; hence the term "born again Christian." In John 3:3, Jesus said, "Truly, truly, I say to you, unless one is born again he cannot see the kingdom of God." Through faith in Christ, you experience a fundamental change in your nature so that you can now coexist with a holy God.

You don't have to pray a formal prayer, walk down an aisle, or perform a ritual. You don't have to be in church. You can be driving in your car, sitting at work, or relaxing in the comfort of your home. You don't have to "clean up your act" first, either. Believe me, you can never be good enough! God doesn't require you to do anything. Just recognize and believe in your heart that the work is already done through the sacrifice of Christ. When you have heard the truth, it is time to make a decision. The apostle Paul writes in 2 Corinthians 6:2 that God has said, "At the acceptable time I listened to you, and on the day of salvation I helped you. Behold, now is 'the acceptable time,' behold, now is 'the day of salvation.'"

None of us know when our time will be up, but we do know that day will come. Heaven is most simply defined as where God is. It is a place of rest, glory, purity, fellowship, and joy in the presence of God. Hell is a place of eternal separation from God and all that is good forever. Hell is a place reserved for people who have been judged and found guilty of unbelief—those who die without trusting Christ as Savior. Christ's desire to rescue you from hell motivated him to die an excruciating death for you. The precise moment you place your faith and trust in the work and person of Jesus Christ is when you are born again and begin an intimate relationship with God through Christ for all eternity.

HEALTH FLASH
TIPS FOR HOLY HOTTIES

Our Wonderful Sense of Sight

With the exception of a few gray hairs (which I only notice every few weeks when I touch up my hair color), my first real sign of aging came to my eyes. I've worn contacts for years for nearsightedness. But, in the last decade, as my prescription for distance got stronger, my near vision was greatly diminished when my contacts were in. At about age forty-eight, I finally could laugh with those who said their arms were too short. I was forced to buy "reading glasses." Other changes were occurring too. My night vision was getting worse and my eyes became more fatigued when I worked at the computer. This would be the first of several failing functions I had once taken for granted and now was seeking advice about.

I chose to have mono-vision lasik surgery a couple years ago. Now I can see perfectly for distance with my left eye and perfectly to read with my right. What I'm left with is my continued night vision problem and a new challenge seeing midrange as clearly as I'd like. Unfortunately, I spend a lot of time using midrange vision on my computer. Being a writer, it's a bit of a challenge some days. So, as usual, I sought the expertise of Dr. Mark Stengler. (Before you're finished with this book, you'll realize why this man is so incredible; he has answers for almost everything!) Here's what I learned about eye health.

Like all areas of our bodies, our eyes need to be supported nutritionally to function optimally. We also need to protect them environmentally from pollutants and ultraviolet rays. That means wearing UV sunglasses whenever we are out in sunlight; this is important for children as well. Whether you are concerned with macular degeneration, poor night vision, cataracts, or eye fatigue, there are many nutritional supplements that can make a big difference over time.

Bilberry, a popular herb also known as European blueberry, is packed with potent antioxidants that reduce cellular damage and improve circulation through the smallest capillaries as well as strengthen those tiny vessel walls. Improved circulation allows valuable nutrients to flow to areas such as the retina of the eye. Visual problems such as those noted above can be prevented and treated with bilberry. The recommended dosage is 160 milligrams twice daily. Eating blueberries regularly can also promote excellent eye health.

Other supplements helpful in dealing with vision include vitamin C, vitamin E, zinc, and ginkgo biloba. Ginkgo is especially effective in treating macular degeneration, diabetic retinopathy, and cataracts.

Taking Action

1. What was the most important truth you gained from this chapter?
2. What changes, if any, do you desire to make related to that truth?
3. What specific thoughts or actions need to be implemented to make those changes?
4. What are your greatest stumbling blocks toward this change?
5. On a scale from one to ten (with ten being the highest) how important is this relative to other needs/changes in your life? Use this scale to help you create an overall action plan when you finish reading this book.

16

What's Your Wheelchair?

As a speaker and radio host, I spend many days considering what meaningful truths I can deposit into the lives of other women—a powerful responsibility and privilege of which I am truly unworthy. God uses me anyway, and the words I speak have truly come from him. It's not unusual though for us "communicators" to sometimes forget to close our mouths and open our ears; we need to be reminded that someone out there might have a message marked "Special Delivery" just for us.

Remembering Who's in Control

Not long ago I took my mom and a friend to a women's outreach event in Coronado, California. The sponsors wanted to make an impact in their community by featuring a motivational Christian speaker who would encourage believers and also speak truth into the hearts of those women who did not know Christ in a personal way. One of the leaders asked me to consider being a future speaker and invited me to experience the format and purpose of their organization by attending.

So there I was in a school gymnasium that brisk December night, getting familiar with their style of ministry so *I* could minister to them most effectively when *I* spoke in the future. Well, *I* quickly realized the evening's purpose was not about what *I* could do for this group. God, in his generosity, was going to feed my soul and nourish my spirit in a unique way. He just needed to slow me down, sit me down, and shut me up long enough to receive his gift from the mouth of another woman!

Renée Bondi—God's Servant

I'd heard very little about the evening's keynote speaker. I knew her name was Renée Bondi. I knew that for some reason she was confined to a wheelchair. I was not prepared for her comedic wit, boundless energy, and contagious joy.

As Renée wheeled onto the stage, I was immediately struck by her radiant smile and the absolute ease with which she moved around by using her partially mobile upper limbs to maneuver her battery-powered chair. Speaking with great enthusiasm and self-effacing humor, she shared the story of a freak sleepwalking (or more accurately "sleep-jumping") accident and the tragedy and blessing of being almost completely paralyzed only weeks before her planned wedding date. Story after story, song after song, I became acutely aware of the indescribable work God can and does do in a surrendered heart.

Renée did not "Pollyanna" her way through this heartbreaking misfortune. She cried out to God with helplessness and sometimes even hopelessness. She assumed her fiancé would never want to marry an invalid. She was wrong. She assumed she would never sing again. She was wrong. She assumed she would never have a child. Again, she was wrong. In fact, she proudly exclaimed from the stage that night, "I not only had a baby, I had completely natural childbirth, and I didn't feel a thing!" The audience broke out in uproarious laughter. I felt a tear well up as I thought about the miracles God had wrought in this woman's life. Why? Simply because he is God, and she was totally dependent upon him.

The Fragility of Life

Watching Renée that night, I realized in a heartbeat any one of us could experience an instantaneous turn of events that would turn our own little world on its head. It is only by God's grace that we experience a new day. He holds all time and eternity in his grasp. In James 4:14 we read, "Yet you do not know what your life will be like tomorrow. You are just a vapor that appears for a little while and then vanishes away." So often though we take every blessing for granted.

I rarely celebrate my ability to walk, run, ski, or dance. I'm more likely to complain about general aches and pains that weren't present a year or two ago. I seldom get excited about the notion of seeing a sunset or even reading a book. Instead, I grumble that my sight just isn't what it used to be and what a pain it is to watch my body slowly flow downhill. I'm trying to slow down my wrinkles, speed up my metabolism, and cover my gray hair as if that will halt the reality of what is *really* going on: my body is deteriorating toward death one cell and one second at a time. It's inevitable!

For Renée, someone must move and massage her limbs daily so they don't curl up in permanent contractures. She must have someone turn her from side to side in bed and inspect her skin for the first sign of pressure sores or abrasions that she will never feel but could lead to massive infections. How frustrating and humiliating it must be to have every private detail of life handled by another person. How completely dependent she must be. Yet how confident and authentic she has become.

Complete Submission

That evening, Renée became a flesh and blood example to me of 1 Peter 5:6–7: "Therefore humble yourselves under the mighty hand of God, that He may exalt you at the proper time, casting all your anxiety on Him, because He cares for you." She admits that, before her accident, she was not sold out to God. She trusted him for her salvation but still had her fists tightly gripped on the control handles of her life. Would she be the same person, sold out for God, surrendered completely, if she had not experienced this accident? Probably not. I wonder: are we the more blessed having our limbs under *our* control . . . or is she, the one who has no control?

We find it difficult to humble ourselves in complete submission when things are going according to our own plans and purposes. Yet James 4:10 says, "Humble yourselves in the presence of the Lord, and He will exalt you." If we seek to be "exalted" in the here and now, that is probably the total measure of our blessing. Webster's defines *exalt* as to "raise in rank" or "glorify." (I don't do that, do I?) Do we have to be some sort of egomaniac to be guilty of seeking personal exaltation? I think not. Each time we set ourselves and our agendas above those of God we are exalting ourselves. When we walk, speak, even minister "in the flesh," we are exalting ourselves. We may have a quiet countenance or subdued personality and still be striving toward personal exaltation without even knowing it. I think we are all guilty of this some of the time. (Perhaps even Renée is at times. But it must be incredibly difficult to live "in the flesh" when you are reminded every single moment of your absolute dependence on God and others.) Those of us who walk and move of our own accord are dependent on God as well; we just don't always realize that fact.

Every single day, we must eat, drink, sleep, and deal with a host of bodily functions that are necessary for our physical survival. God didn't have to create us with these demanding human bodies, but he did. The older (or sicker) we get, the greater the reminder that we have little control over this corporeal existence. We are shackled and dependent on God's provision. Without this failing flesh, would *any* of us surrender and lean into God in total submission? Probably not. But because there is so much in this life out of our control, we realize we need the One who has all things in his control.

A Wake-up Call

What is your wheelchair? What will force you out of the driver's seat and put God in complete control? What will put you in a wheelchair of sorts that forces you to realize the truth of what God says in Isaiah 55:8–9?

> "For My thoughts are not your thoughts,
> Nor are your ways My ways," declares the LORD.
> "For as the heavens are higher than the earth,
> So are My ways higher than your ways
> And My thoughts than your thoughts."

I believe with all my heart that this Scripture is true, but I certainly don't always live it. Some years ago, I got a little wake-up call of sorts that impacted me significantly. It happened on one of my busy days. Rushing out of the house, coffee cup and briefcase in hand, I was stretching the limits of efficient time management by trying to get to a business meeting seventy minutes away—I had sixty minutes to get there on time.

The freeway traffic was flowing fast for a Monday morning. As I finished a call on my cell phone and placed my right hand back on the steering wheel, an unusual heaviness fell into my hands; the steering wheel had come completely off the column! My first thought was, *I'm going to get hurt today!*

I tried in vain to replace the steering wheel, but it seemed as if time stood still. No control! Since I couldn't brake, I kept my foot on the gas to avoid being rear-ended by another driver, wondering exactly where my car was going to end up.

My heart was pounding as I clearly realized I had no options. My life and safety were not in my power, and my heart cried out silently to the Lord, "God, I can't do anything. It's up to you." Miraculously, I cleared the first lane and then the second. I don't know where all the cars were for those split seconds, but they seemed to disappear. It was as if angels were guiding me across that treacherous route.

Still traveling at about fifty miles per hour, my car crossed smoothly onto the left shoulder, the front tire barely skimming the concrete safety curb. At that moment, I slammed on the brakes and came to a screeching halt, the barrier stabilizing my car and preventing me from spinning into the rush hour traffic.

Suddenly, I became aware of the loud whoosh of cars passing me at seventy miles per hour. Dropping the steering wheel into my lap, I raised my shaking hands and yelled, "Hey, everybody, slow down. Don't you know? You're really not in control of anything! You're not going anywhere unless God lets you!"

God had captured my attention that morning. I was shaken by the possibility that it could have been my very last day on earth. Had I lived it to the fullest? Did my life really have purpose or meaning? Was I wasting too much time and energy on things that had little lasting value? I realized I had been living life out of control and without focus for far too long. That day I made a lifetime commitment—to live with balance and purpose. And I did . . . for a while. I still try, but I must admit that experience seems more like a scene from a movie than the adrenaline-pounding occurrence it really was. How can I keep that sense of God's control at the top of my mind every day, not so I live out of fear but rather with a reality of eternity while I travel this temporal road of life?

Maintaining a godly (God-obsessed) perspective is difficult. We work to live and live to work. We strive and scramble to pay bills, meet goals, and find some sense of accomplishment and purpose. In the flesh, we are driven to fulfill the desires of the flesh (and those aren't necessarily sinful), but as believers, we are new creations with a holy God taking residence in our very spirit drawing us to himself. I see a different joy, purpose, and surrender in Renée Bondi's life; it's as obvious as her wheelchair. She has a constant reminder of her dependence that keeps her mentally, emotionally, and spiritually shackled to God's power. Must *we* live in a wheelchair to have that kind of daily perspective? Perhaps. That is why I said earlier, it may be difficult to see accurately who really has the greater blessing. I'm thinking God's "higher ways" are being lived out right now in his sweet servant Renée.

I've pondered several times on the words of the apostle Paul in Philippians 1:21: "For to me, to live is Christ and to die is gain." I'm not ready to die. I don't think I'm afraid, but I have so much to do and so many things I want to experience. I don't want to leave my husband or children just yet. If I saw all things with complete accuracy, I'd be banging on the gates of heaven, begging, "Jesus take me now; this place down here is nuts!" But I see things from my limited vantage point.

In the meantime, God allows both gentle and sometimes not so gentle reminders about our fragile "vaporlike" existence—

steering wheels that fall off on the freeway, September 11, the passing of a friend or loved one. We are impacted for a season, but then that human and very resilient spirit kicks in and we move back into a sense of power and control.

My gentle reminder on December 7, 2003, came via an angel who sang from a wheelchair in a middle school gym nineteen years after losing total control of her body. She sang to the Lord, songs that nourished her soul and expressed the joy and fear of being totally dependent and surrendered to him. Right after her accident, she couldn't sing at all, but God exalted her humble, broken body. Despite what the doctors said was impossible, God allowed her diaphragm to expand enough to push out the sweet voice she so loved to use for him. It had been her greatest joy to be a choral director. She is once again . . . at her church and wherever she speaks. Renée led us in a song that night. I can't even remember the words. I just kept thinking, *Must it take a wheelchair to humble ourselves so completely that God exalts us in such a way?*

I've been asking myself, "What is *my* wheelchair?" The "disabilities" I experience are of the mind and heart, my traumas most often self-induced. I'd pray for a real "wheelchair," but that's awfully scary. Until then, I suppose I will simply ponder . . . and wonder what it must be like to be exalted by the Most High God.

HEALTH FLASH
TIPS FOR HOLY HOTTIES

Outsmarting Osteoporosis

I have a confession. Despite my medical and fitness experience, I have often ignored issues like osteoporosis. I assumed that my decades of exercise and decent nutrition would certainly insulate *me* from this "old lady" disease. Well, I'm not going to put my head in the sand anymore. I'm hearing creaks and cracks I never heard before; I'm feeling tweaks and twinges that are new and quite distressing. There are things going on beneath the surface that I can't see and most likely can't feel, but they are happening nonetheless. One of those things is bone loss. Statistics reveal that one out of two women over fifty will have an osteoporosis-related fracture in their lifetime. I've got some facts and advice that are better taken now than later, because one of the hardest things to reverse is severe bone loss. So let's get "bone healthy" together.

Bone is living tissue that is constantly breaking down and reforming. It is estimated that we have a completely new skeleton every seven years, but if we're not getting the right nutrients or enough exercise, the frame we have tomorrow will be inferior to the one we have today. We must address good bone health from childhood on.

Osteoporosis means "porous bone." It begins without any signs or symptoms. Over time, women will find themselves "shrinking" as the spongy trabecular bone of the vertebrae start to crumble and collapse one millimeter at a time. Some people with severe osteoporosis suffer a fracture by simply bumping into something. The strength of all our bones is greatly influenced by hormones, immobilization, and the use of certain medications such as prednisone. Cortical bone is the hard, protective covering of the bone found in the long bones of the arms and legs. Its strength is influenced most by minerals such as calcium and magnesium. In addition, collagen is an important protein that works to provide a kind of reinforcement so that bones are strong, yet flexible; it also helps minerals and other proteins to bind together to form new bone.

Risk Factors

Many factors increase your risk of osteoporosis. While a bone-density study is the best and recommended way to accurately assess your risk, these factors may motivate you toward that end. Don't assume if you're not a super high risk you have no risk. That is simply not true. You may want to circle the factors that pertain to you to help you assess your personal level or risk.

1. Female
2. Over fifty or postmenopausal (haven't had a period for more than twelve months)
3. Caucasian or Asian
4. Family history of osteoporosis
5. No full-term pregnancies
6. History of stress fractures
7. Late menses or irregular periods or ovulation
8. Thin or small body frame or low body fat
9. Diabetes, anorexia, bulimia, kidney or liver disease
10. Medications: anticonvulsants, prednisone, heparin, methotrexate, lithium, antacids, excessive thyroid hormone medication
11. Diet high in caffeine, alcohol, sugar, phosphate (soda), sodium, or animal protein
12. Poor gastric absorption
13. Smoking
14. Inactivity
15. Low hormone levels

Whew. What a list. Obviously there are some things completely out of your control. But there are a few, such as diet and lifestyle habits, that you can do something about!

The Hormone Connection

According to Dr. Stengler, if low hormones and diminished bone density are both present, natural progesterone either used by itself or in addition to bio-identical estrogen is recommended in treating or preventing osteoporosis. In severe cases, growth hormone is being taken more seriously as a therapy as it appears to stimulate bone growth.

Researchers have also found an interesting connection between an imbalanced immune system and bone loss—one more reason to eat and live for optimal health.

> Dr. Stengler has a "moo-ving" fact he encouraged me to share with you. He writes: "Powerful media advertisements by the dairy industry have led people to believe that cow's milk is ambrosia to the bones. While dairy milk does contain about 300 mg of calcium per 8 ounce serving, the calcium is not well absorbed. Considering that milk is one of the most common food allergens, high in phosphorous (which causes calcium excretion) and contaminated with hormones (unless organic), I do not recommend it as a primary source of calcium."[1]

Conventional treatment for osteoporosis is most often the synthetic hormone Premarin or another estrogen product alone or in combination with synthetic progesterone. In addition, Alendronate (the most popular brand—Fosamax) is a nonhormonal drug that has been shown to increase bone density. The most common side effect is irritation and ulceration of the esophagus.

Strong Bones the Natural Way

There are several natural ways to stimulate strong bones and prevent osteoporosis.

1. Exercising—both weight bearing and strength training—is beneficial.

2. Eating foods that support bone growth, such as:
   a. Vegetables—which promote alkalinity
   b. Essential fatty acids
   c. Healthy proteins—less from animal sources (it will be interesting to see how the high protein diets will impact aging baby boomers in years to come)
   d. Moderate consumption of soy
3. Reducing stress; when cortisol is elevated for long periods, it leads to breakdown of bone tissue.
4. Bone-specific supplements are beneficial: 1,200 milligrams a day are recommended for menopausal women. The best sources are calcium citrate, citrate-malate, aspartate, or gluconate. These supplements are best taken with meals. Magnesium at 500 milligrams a day and vitamin D at 400 to 1,200 IU are also essential for bone health.
5. Taking vitamin K in doses of 150 to 500 milligrams per day has been shown to be helpful.

Most experts agree that the best approach to treatment and prevention starts with working with a quality physician and basing your health treatment on accurate test results.

My ministry partner and I once created a David Letterman-like list of why women get depressed.

#10 No chocolate

 #9 You ate too much chocolate

 #8 No money to go shopping

 #7 Money to shop . . . nothing fits

 #6 Nobody remembered your birthday

 #5 Everyone remembered your birthday AND your age

 #4 Your kids won't allow you any time to yourself

 #3 Your kids are grown and don't have time for you

 #2 Three-way mirrors

 #1 Seeing yourself in a swimsuit in a three-way mirror

Taking Action

1. What was the most important truth you gained from this chapter?
2. What changes, if any, do you desire to make related to that truth?
3. What specific thoughts or actions need to be implemented to make those changes?
4. What are your greatest stumbling blocks toward this change?
5. On a scale from one to ten (with ten being the highest) how important is this relative to other needs/changes in your life? Use this scale to help you create an overall action plan when you finish reading this book.

17

Feeling Down? Look Up!

I never used to get depressed. In fact, for years I didn't understand how people could get stuck in even a mild funk. It just wasn't me. Then, more recently, in dealing with rebellious daughters and other challenging "stuff," I started to get a glimpse of what others go through.

Sometimes laughing about the things that get us down helps. Laughter helps us cope by releasing wonderful chemicals into our brain. But laughter alone is rarely enough. Some days just getting through the emotional ups and downs of menopause seems like more than I can bear, and I wonder why I'm feeling blue for no apparent reason. I know I'm not alone. Many friends and acquaintances close to my age feel low now and then too.

These days I find that even little inconveniences get me down. Getting through the lines at the grocery store becomes an incredible irritation because I absolutely *hate* standing in lines. I feel like a military general trying to analyze which one will move the fastest. Inevitably, there's a glitch in my calculations. The cashier decides to go on a break as my turn approaches. Or the register runs out of paper. And there are the unforeseen disasters like the woman with a bazillion coupons. It's always something. Perhaps God is *still* trying to teach me patience.

Nevertheless, there *are* times when waiting in line is worthwhile: waiting for a busy jeweler to help you pick out your engagement ring; waiting to hear your favorite musical group or to see a Broadway play. And some things you'd just as soon wait for *forever*: your annual dental hygiene appointment, your audit with an IRS agent, and most of all . . . your turn to die.

Embracing Life

My friend Marita shared a lot with me about waiting to die. In the process, she helped me celebrate with joy this season of menopause that I am experiencing. She told me once, "We're all in line to die. Most of us just don't know when it will happen." When she found out she had terminal cancer, she realized that she had been abruptly "bumped to the front of the line." She said, "I'm battling this thing and I'm going to fight for a number two or three position in that line as long as I can. But, at some point, we all get to the front and have to jump off!"

Marita made some decisions about the perspective she would have during her fight with cancer. Early on, she decided that she would officially declare her weekends "cancer-free" zones. From 4:00 on Friday afternoon until 8:00 on Monday morning, she did not discuss her cancer, talk with doctors, or worry about her next treatment. This was not an act of denial;

it was Marita's way of placing healthy boundaries over this menacing invader. She absolutely refused to allow her cancer to consume every detail of her life.

How do we put boundaries around our perspective in dealing with the tough issues of life? Without diminishing the reality that hormones do intensify our emotions, we still need to embrace the fact that every emotion we experience is a direct result of our perspective—or more specifically our beliefs.

If you believe that you are "over-the-hill" or no longer attractive, your emotions will match that belief and you will feel "less than" the woman you once were. *That* is a lie. Embrace the truth. You are "more than" you used to be. Stop defining yourself by the wrinkles and sags and start seeing the depth of character all these years of living have cultivated in your very soul! Celebrate every breath you take, every day the Lord has gifted you on this planet. You never know which one will be your last.

A Heavenly Perspective

In talking about death, I asked Marita if she had any fears. She said that she knew she was going to heaven and shared what one of her friends had told her: "Marita, when you get to the edge of the cliff between life and death, just remember . . . look up!" Marita added that the hard part was leaving those she loved behind. She wished that someone who had gone before her could come back and tell her what it was like. In reality, someone *had* gone before and *did* come back to tell her. His name is Jesus. He told his friends in John 14, "There is plenty of room for you in my Father's home. If that weren't so, would I have told you that I'm on my way to get a room ready for you?" (personal paraphrase).

Over time, Marita began to see what Jesus meant by those words. She spent time reading the Bible and studying so that she would have a clearer perspective about life. She came to realize that we spend such a short time on earth and forever in heaven. That truth gave Marita a deeply comforting perspective as she continued her battle with cancer. Today she completely understands—because she recently met Jesus face-to-face. Marita lost her battle with cancer but won a victory over death!

Why do we fear the unknown? We fear because our understanding is limited.

When we see our lives through eternal eyes, "we groan, longing to be clothed with our heavenly dwelling . . . [for we] know that as long as we are at home in the body we are away from the Lord" (2 Cor. 5:2, 6 NIV). Just think—despite our deteriorating bodies, one day we will have a glorified body when Christ returns. Wow! No more wrinkles, no more sags, no more hot flashes! Now *that* is an important perspective to focus on when we're feeling down.

I learned so much from Marita in the short time I knew her. I learned about friendship, hope, and love. I learned that I have a choice about the perspective I will choose to embrace each day. During her battle, Marita would wake each morning, breathe in the fresh air, look out at the sunrise, and celebrate that God had given her the gift of one more day. Then, before she turned out the light at night, she pulled out her journal and wrote down five things she was grateful for. Marita gave me a "grateful journal" last year. Today I wrote the five things I am most grateful for:

1. I am grateful that nothing can shatter hope.
2. I am grateful that nothing can corrode faith.
3. I am grateful that nothing can kill friendship.

4. I am grateful that friends like Marita will last forever because . . .

5. Jesus died that we may live eternally. For *that* I am most grateful!

A friend of mine forwarded an email she received that illustrates the importance of perspective in the realities of life. Like Marita's story, it touched my heart and helped me to see my life with fresh eyes. This is how it read:

Recently I overheard a father and daughter in their last moments together at the airport. They had announced her plane departure and, standing near the security gate, they hugged and he said, "I love you. I wish you enough."

She said, "Daddy, our life together has been more than enough. Your love is all I ever needed. I wish you enough, too, Daddy." They kissed and she left. He walked over toward the window where I was seated. I could see he wanted and needed to cry.

I tried not to intrude on his privacy, but he welcomed me in by asking, "Did you ever say good-bye to someone knowing it would be forever?" "Yes, I have," I replied. Saying that brought back memories I had of expressing my love and appreciation for all my Dad had done for me. Recognizing that his days were limited, I took the time to tell him face-to-face how much he meant to me. So I knew what this man was experiencing.

"Forgive me for asking, but why is this a forever good-bye?" I asked.

"I am old and she lives much too far away. I have challenges ahead and the reality is, the next trip back will be for my funeral," he said.

"When you were saying good-bye I heard you say, 'I wish you enough.' May I ask what that means?"

He began to smile. "That's a wish that has been handed down from generation to generation in my family. My parents used to say it to everyone. And now, my daughter and I always say it when we part." He paused for a moment and, looking up as if trying to remember, he smiled even more and continued:

"When we said 'I wish you enough,' we were wanting the other person to have a life filled with just enough good things to sustain them," he continued and then turning toward me recited it from memory . . .

I wish you enough sun to keep your attitude bright.

I wish you enough rain to appreciate the sun more.

I wish you enough happiness to keep your spirit alive.

I wish you enough pain that the smallest joys in life appear much bigger.

I wish you enough gain to satisfy your wanting.

I wish you enough loss to appreciate all that you possess.

I wish you enough "Hello's" to get you through the final "Good-bye."

If this elderly man and my friend Marita could have such hopeful and grounded perspectives in their last years of life, I am sure we can do the same through each of our daily challenges. Sometimes, all we need is a moment to check our negative perspective at the door and adopt an accurate and more hopeful one.

Living in the moment is essential to finding contentment. Marita taught me so much about that truth. When I experience the emotional roller coaster of my "menopause moments" or wake in the still of the night wondering who turned the heat on high and realize I *am* the furnace, I try my best to remember Marita's words of wisdom and an old man's "wish you enough" perspective. As I struggle to calm my estrogen-starved nerves or get back to sleep, I take a few moments to record a few things I am thankful for in the journal of my mind knowing each moment, each day, is a gift. Will I embrace all that it offers and rejoice or will I grumble and complain? It's my choice. It's yours. Let's choose to rejoice together. "I wish you enough."

HEALTH FLASH

TIPS FOR HOLY HOTTIES

Dealing with Depression

Menopause doesn't necessarily make women moody, but some studies suggest that depression may be more likely during this time. Some of the explanations include:

1. Symptoms may drive mood swings.
2. Hot flashes and night sweats can disrupt the ever-so-important sleep cycle causing irritability, poor concentration, and anxiety.
3. Decreasing estrogen and progesterone levels can trigger biochemical changes in the brain that may result in depression.
4. Some women may have an unhealthy perspective about midlife and its issues.
5. Stressful life events, such as elderly parents needing care, grown children leaving home, and career or relationship changes, can trigger depressive episodes.

In *Your Menopause, Your Menotype*, Dr. Stengler states:

We know that estrogen helps maintain the neurotransmitter serotonin, which is important for our "good moods." Other key hormones, like progesterone, DHEA, cortisol, thyroid and others are involved in balancing the brain's electrical activity. We also know that synthetic hormones can actually trigger depression. Fortunately, we can usually reverse this situation by converting the woman to a more natural approach.[1]

Obviously, you must get to the root of a problem to address it effectively. If you have a clogged drain, there is no point going out and buying a new sink. You must "get the stuff out" of the drain. But so often the moods and even depression associated with menopause are multifaceted and require a look in several directions. If the issue is emotional or psychological, you will want to make sure your perspective is accurate and grounded in God's Word. No matter *why* you are feeling as you do, don't neglect the powerful encouragement in James 1:5: "But if any of you lacks wisdom, let him ask of God, who gives to all generously and without reproach, and it will be given to him."

Whenever I am seeking answers, this is one of the first verses the Holy Spirit brings to my mind. I pray that God would give me the wisdom to find the right answers. (And sometimes even to *ask* the right questions first!) I also pray for those who are helping me such as my doctors or mentors. Never underestimate the power of prayer grounded in accurately applied biblical promises. And this is one of them!

As I addressed in chapters 7, 8, and 9, nothing takes the place of getting back to basics in generating overall health and well-being. In addition to eating healthy whole foods for maximum energy, some key nutrients essential to good mental health include the powerful omega-3s (see chapter 2), B vitamins, and amino acids (found in protein sources). Additionally, exercise has been shown to have a positive effect on both moods and depression. If you are not getting purposeful exercise almost every day, take action, and just do it!

Beyond healthy habits, there are certainly many natural and healthful ways to address the moodiness or depression associated with menopause. First and foremost, review the natural approaches outlined in the Health Flash segments of this book. Many natural herbal therapies such as black cohosh not only diminish hot flashes but also other symptoms associated with your fluctuating hormones, including the blues.

Despite some recent reports to the contrary, Dr. Stengler still feels confident that Saint-John's-wort can be an effective herb in dealing specifically with depression associated with menopause. Other helpful herbs that enhance relaxation and promote sleep, such as valerian, chamomile, 5HTP, SAMe, and melatonin, can be helpful depending on the cause of your depression. If you are irritable due to lack of sleep, getting enough sleep (perhaps with some natural help) may be the answer.

Always make sure you have one health advocate who is aware of all aspects of your health. I highly recommend finding a qualified naturopathic physician in your area. A professional who can see the whole picture of your health and help you find the most natural remedies possible is a great asset to you now and in the years to come. While many practitioners in the area of natural health are New Age, I have found more and more Christians entering this field. It's worth the search!

Journaling the ups and downs of your moods and bouts with depression can be very helpful. Try to draw some correlations to lack of sleep, the weather, what you are eating, the severity of your menopause symptoms, and so forth. With your doctor's approval, try one new herbal or supplemental remedy at a time for a period of at least two to three weeks so you can determine what kind of impact it is making. Simply writing your thoughts and feelings can be very cathartic. Pray through the issues that bring you down and whenever possible talk them out with a trusted friend or your spouse. Don't let your pride or your desire to protect others keep you from the benefit of sharing your difficulties. That's what part of life is about—loving each other through the pain.

My friend Carol, a popular local news anchor, had a breakdown on the air many years ago. She struggled with depression her entire adult life. When she spoke at our Women of Purpose outreach event, we were blown away by how many women commented on their battles with depression. She helped the women get over the stigma of depression and reminded us it is impossible to get help if we don't let someone know we have a problem.

If you discover that your depression is due to a chemical imbalance, don't be afraid to try medications that may help. As Carol discovered the hard way, her brain would default to a "tilt" setting again and again if she didn't stay consistently on her medication. She shared an important perspective I think many Christians fail to realize when we grapple with the issue of being "dependent" on a drug. To better grasp this, let me ask you: Would you take insulin if you were a diabetic? Would you use an inhaler if you had asthma? Would you take medication for high blood pressure? Of course you would. Well, your brain is an organ. It can become diseased or malfunction just like other organs can. Don't overspiritualize the need to take medication for depression . . . even if it means taking it for a lifetime. Just thank God that medical technology has increased to the point where there is something available!

If needed, by all means seek godly Christian counsel through a well-respected therapist or psychologist. Seeking help is never a sign of weakness. But it is foolish to isolate yourself and try to deal with these things on your own. You need to be vulnerable enough that those around you know you are hurting. Sharing your burden with another human being can help lift the weight of depression.

Taking Action

1. What was the most important truth you gained from this chapter?
2. What changes, if any, do you desire to make related to that truth?
3. What specific thoughts or actions need to be implemented to make those changes?
4. What are your greatest stumbling blocks toward this change?
5. On a scale from one to ten (with ten being the highest) how important is this relative to other needs/changes in your life? Use this scale to help you create an overall action plan when you finish reading this book.

18

Living with Purpose . . . Leaving a Legacy

I am twice my oldest daughter's age. Yesterday *I* was twenty-six . . . now *she* is. I blinked my eyes and whoa—I'm fifty-plus. I still have hopes and dreams. I look to the future expectantly, desiring to be all God has called me to be. I see myself living out the movie of my life—the young heroine conquering life's challenges. And I am forever young in my mind despite the fact that the calendar and mirror argue with *my* reality.

It seems like a few short years ago I was having my first child. I held her in my arms and wondered if I would ever measure up as a mother. It's hard to believe I'm already a grandmother with hot flashes. Where did the years go? More important, how will I spend the rest?

A Personal Eulogy

At one time or another, you've probably been encouraged to write your own eulogy as an exercise in exploring your life purpose. You know the drill—write what you would want someone to say about you at your funeral. Actually, it's a pretty good idea. Writing what you *want* said helps you take an inventory of how close you are to your objective.

My pastor, Tim Scott, attended the funeral of a minister who had been an old family friend. He was blown away by all the wonderful things that were shared as one person after another conveyed how this incredible man had impacted their lives. Pastor Scott was so moved by the consistency and authenticity of this friend's life that he became inspired to not only think about his own eulogy but, more important, to *live* his eulogy. In other words, to invest each day in people as if it were his last.

I encourage you to finish the prompters below regarding how you want to be remembered right now. You know if you don't do it now, you'll probably never do it. So, how about investing a few minutes in this important exercise? At my funeral, I want others to say . . .

She was a

She made a difference through

She touched my life by

Please don't allow thinking about your funeral to be a downer. If you know Jesus Christ as your Savior, you know that the years after your funeral will indeed be the best to come. Yet this side of heaven you need the right perspective to ensure your remaining earthbound years are vital and fulfilling. You can be sure that the *wrong* perspective is thinking that your fading youth is something to be mourned, that you have missed the most important opportunities life has to offer, or that you have nothing left to give. Accept the past as past and live abundantly in the present. Accept your aging body with grace. You can slow the process, but you can't stop it. So get over it and get on with it!

A Foundation of Truth

We need to realize that even though the body withers, wisdom can abound. I believe we can make the most profound investments into others' lives in these "mature" years. I love what Dr. Maryann Rosenthal, a clinical psychologist, says about aging and wisdom: "One thing younger women can't have that we *do* have is experience and wisdom. We need to realize that wisdom is sexy. So, flaunt your wisdom!"

In the book of Titus, the older women are called to encourage the younger women to love their husbands, to love their children, and to be mature and sensible in all areas of life. But to do so requires a strong foundation of truth—the truth that is found when we filter all of our life experiences and actions through the grid of biblical certainty.

Ask yourself these questions: "What does God's Word say about my life?" "What does it say is the 'most important' thing?" "What does it tell me about finding fulfillment and joy?" The Bible says "the truth will set us free" (John 8:32), but if we don't know that truth intimately, we won't know true freedom; nor will we be able to pass it on to others.

First Things First . . . The One Thing

Years ago, I was a corporate marketing manager and had the privilege of teaching Stephen Covey's *The Seven Habits of Highly Effective People* to the employees of our Fortune 100 company. In his book, he made a statement that really made me think. He said something like this: "What one thing could you do (if you did it on a regular basis) that would make the biggest, most positive impact in your life?"

Think about that question: What *one* thing? The first thing that came to my mind was what Jesus said in Matthew 6:33: "But seek first His kingdom and His righteousness, and all these things will be added to you." If life is to have true meaning, purpose, and joy, we have to put first things first. As believers, we *know* what that is. It is God, his Word, his plan, and his purpose. Yet too often we seek our own desires and gratification first.

Living with purpose requires that we not only know truth but apply it effectively to our lives. To do so, we need to discover the "One Thing" that is most essential in *each* dimension of our lives and give it time and attention until dynamic change has been achieved.

A few years ago, I spoke on this very subject to a group of women. We identified six key life categories, their underlying principles, and Scripture to help us choose the "One Thing" that was most vital in that area of our lives at that time. It was a powerful exercise that I will pass on to you below. We've dealt with each dimension in at least one chapter of this book. Now let's take a little journey toward finding clearer purpose. Then we will be better prepared to leave a legacy that will far outlast our meager stint here on planet Earth.

Six Key Life Categories

#1—The Physical Dimension

PRINCIPLES

1. Your body is your only vehicle for life.

2. You are what you eat.
3. If you don't "use it" you'll "lose it."

SCRIPTURE

[Offer] your bodies as living sacrifices, holy and pleasing to God—this is your spiritual act of worship.

Romans 12:1 NIV

You know the importance of your health and how it impacts every area of your life. We covered this dimension in some detail in chapters 7, 8, and 9. Consider your answers at the end of those chapters.

QUESTION

What one thing will *you* act on that will make the biggest difference in your physical body and health this year?

#2—The Material Dimension

PRINCIPLE

You can't take it with you.

SCRIPTURE

For this reason I say to you, do not worry about your life, as to what you will eat; nor for your body, as to what you will put on. For life is more than food, and the body more than clothing.

Luke 12:22

Stuff . . . stuff . . . stuff. We addressed the issue of our material dimension in chapter 15, "You Can't Take It with You." What in that chapter helped you the most? How is this area of your life doing right now?

QUESTION

What one thing will *you* act on that will make the biggest difference in your material dimension this year?

#3—The Mental Dimension

PRINCIPLE

You are what you think.

SCRIPTURE

Do not be conformed to this world, but be transformed by the renewing of your mind.

Romans 12:2

In chapter 4, "The 'Change' That Transforms Your Life," we discussed the incredible power of the human mind. We also discussed how God's Word is living and active, sharper than any two-edged sword. We are transformed by the renewing of our minds. What most impacted you about that chapter? How do you need to renew your mind?

QUESTION

What one thing will *you* act on that will make the biggest difference in your mental dimension this year?

#4—The Emotional Dimension

PRINCIPLE

Feelings—both good and bad—are a direct result of what you believe.

SCRIPTURE

For the mouth speaks out of that which fills the heart.

Matthew 12:34

Women are "feeling" creatures. We often wear our emotions on our sleeves and make decisions based on "gut feelings." Many times, however, our emotions are not reliable indicators. When we have faulty beliefs or if our hormones are out of control, we need to use what we *know*, not what we feel, to govern our decisions and actions. We have covered many of these principles about having an accurate perspective and belief system throughout the book. Think about negative emotions you are experiencing that are impacting your life. Are there lies attached to those emotions?

QUESTION
What one thing will *you* act on that will make the biggest difference in your emotional dimension this year?

#5—The Relational Dimension

PRINCIPLE
Human beings are designed for relationship.

SCRIPTURE
The LORD God said, "It is not good for the man to be alone; I will make a helper suitable for him."

Genesis 2:18

We need intimate connections with people (not just mates). But people can and do hurt us. Shall we love anyway? How have your past relationships negatively impacted your current ones? What relationship is causing you the most pain right now? Realizing that you cannot control another's feelings or actions, what *can* you do to impact that relationship in a positive way? Whether you are single or married, I hope you read chapters 12, 13, and 14 as they contain important principles about how we are designed relationally for both God and human connection.

QUESTION

What one thing will *you* act on that will make the biggest difference in your relational dimension this year?

#6—The Spiritual Dimension

PRINCIPLE

We were designed for the ultimate relationship—intimacy with God.

SCRIPTURE

And you shall love the Lord your God with all your heart, and with all your soul, and with all your mind, and with all your strength.

Mark 12:30

When Jesus was asked what the most important commandment was, he answered with the Scripture verse above. Throughout Scripture, we are taught consistently to "put first things first." Even as you look back at the other five dimensions, you will find that if you leave this most important principle out, you will have a huge gap in your soul and spirit. In fact, it is my contention that if this becomes our primary and sole purpose, all the rest will fall together.

QUESTION

What one thing will *you* act on that will make the biggest difference in your spiritual dimension this year?

I have no clue what you wrote that would most deeply impact your spiritual dimension. Perhaps you decided you needed to pray more, study the Bible, go to church regularly, or serve in ministry. I propose to you that if any of your answers were more about "doing" than "being," you are on the wrong track. I am no theologian, and I'm not even near where I want to be in this dimension. But I do know that loving the Lord with all my heart, mind, soul, and strength is about falling deeply in love with the One who *is* love.

When we feel alone, lost, fearful, or anxious we have forgotten "whose" we are. If we could accurately see in the spiritual dimension, we would never go to those places again. I believe the reason Paul could say, "For to me, to live is Christ and to die is gain" (Phil. 1:21), was because he did have mature spiritual sight. He had fallen deeply in love with Christ and could no longer see through the world's lenses. He wasn't in love because he served, prayed, wrote letters, and preached. He preached, wrote letters, prayed, and served because he was in love.

In God's Presence

Think about the first time you fell deeply in love. Your heart and mind were constantly drawn to that special person. You spent as much time with him as life would allow. You thought about him continuously and found endless ways to make his day special. You shared your every thought and the deepest secrets of your heart with him. It is no different with God. You get to know him by studying his Word. You fall in love with him as you realize the depth of his unconditional love for you. James 4:8 says, "Draw near to God and He will draw near to you." Draw near to him by practicing his presence and pouring out your heart in prayer. He is listening. This is what my pastor, Tim Scott, says about intimacy with God:

Love for God results in intimacy. And, intimacy combined with the truth from God's Word applied to our life, results in victory. Love is our motivator and dependency on God is our power. Let your love for God and His for you become your primary motivator in all you do. This focus will ultimately transform your life as you build a strong and unshakeable identity in Christ.[1]

Brother Lawrence

Two books profoundly impacted my life this year. The first, *The Practice of the Presence of God*, was sent to me as a gift by my literary agent, Chip MacGregor. It is based on the life and perspectives of a sixteenth-century French lay monk named Brother Lawrence. This unique man made it his life's mission to continually practice the presence of God every moment of the day. You might think, *Easy for him; he was a monk with nothing else to do but dwell on God.* But that's not so. He had full responsibilities that kept him busy and challenged. Yet he chose to take every task, every conversation, and do it "as unto the Lord." Over time, his habit of practicing the presence of God became so ingrained that he no longer had to work at it. When facing extreme adversity, Brother Lawrence once said, "It no longer matters to me what I may do, or what I may suffer, provided that I remain lovingly united to His will, which is my only concern."

I so love God and am thankful for his gift of eternal life. Seeing Mel Gibson's movie *The Passion of the Christ* recently moved me to unstoppable tears. However, on a day-to-day basis, I struggle like most people to be tuned in to God's presence constantly. On several occasions, I've made it my "purpose of the day" to do a temperature check of sorts each hour and consider if I've been aware of God in that time frame. I'm appalled when two or three hours fly by and I forget my purpose in the busyness of living. After reading of Brother Lawrence's practice, I even made little strips of paper that said PPG (Practice the Presence of God) and posted them everywhere I frequently looked. It didn't help as much as I had hoped. But I am still impacted deeply by this concept and will continue my pursuit. For I truly believe that this practice, coupled with deep study of God's Word, will do more to transform us into godly women than anything else.

Here is a description of Brother Lawrence's method of practicing the presence of God moment to moment in his own words:

So filled as I was with the grandeur of this infinite Being, I went to enclose myself in the place which obedience had marked out for me—which was the kitchen. There, alone, after having made provision for everything connected with my duties, I spent all my remaining time in prayer, both before and after work. At the beginning of my duties, I said to God with a son-like trust, "My God, since You are with me, and since it is Your will that I should apply my mind to these outward things, I pray that You will give me the grace to remain with You and keep company with You. But so that my work may be better, Lord, work with me; receive my work and possess all my affections." Finally, during my work, I continued to speak to Him in a familiar way, offering Him my little services, and asking for His grace. At the end of my work, I examined how I had done it, and if I found any good in it, I thanked God. If I noticed errors, I asked His forgiveness for them, and without becoming discouraged, I resolved to change and began anew to remain with God as if I had never strayed. So, by picking myself up after my falls, and by doing many little acts of faith and love, I came to a state in which it would be as difficult for me not to think of God as it had been difficult to accustom myself of thinking of Him at the beginning.[2]

I am ashamed and humbled when looking at my own life, knowing that another human being could so unselfishly give himself up purely for the love of God. For Brother Lawrence, his means of going to God was to do everything out of love for him. It was God, not the work, that he considered. He understood that God, having need of nothing, considers only the love that accompanies our work. It is said that this simple yet deeply spiritual man admired nothing, was astonished by nothing, and feared nothing. His stability of soul came from knowing God in a profoundly intimate way. Hearing of such reckless abandon in our times is rare. Yet I was encouraged to find a more modern man who had been greatly influenced by saints such as Brother Lawrence and wrote powerful truths only decades ago.

A. W. Tozer

The second book challenging my mind and pulling at my heart this year is A. W. Tozer's *The Pursuit of God*. Tozer was the pastor of Southside Alliance Church in Chicago for thirty-one years. He wrote until his death in 1963. Like Brother Lawrence, he was sold out to God. He was also passionate about calling serious believers back to a deeper level of connection with God. While both these books are written in a less than modern vernacular, I found the concepts well grounded in biblical truth. Please allow me to share a few of my favorite excerpts from *The Pursuit of God*. You will see the common thread these thoughts share with *The Practice of the Presence of God*. I'm quite sure God didn't allow me to read these this year by accident. Tozer writes about faith:

Faith is occupied with the Object upon which it rests and pays no attention to itself at all. While we are looking at God we do not see ourselves—blessed riddance. While we look

268

at Christ, the very things we have so long been trying to do will be getting done within us.

Now, if faith is the gaze of the heart at God, and if this gaze is but the raising of the inward eyes to meet the all-seeing eyes of God, then it follows that it is one of the easiest things possible to do. It would be like God to make the most vital thing easy and place it within the range of possibility for the weakest and poorest of us.[3]

He also writes about gazing on God:

Many have found the secret of which I speak. Without giving much thought to what is going on within them, they constantly practice this habit of inwardly gazing upon God. Even when they are compelled to withdraw their conscious attention in order to engage in earthly affairs, there is within them a secret communion always going on. When the habit of inwardly gazing Godward becomes fixed within us, we shall be ushered onto a new level of spiritual life more in keeping with the promises of God and the mood of the New Testament. The triune God will be our dwelling place even while our feet walk the low road of simple duty here among men.[4]

Tozer concludes his book in essence saying that it is not *what* we do that matters to God; it is *why* we do it. For God, motive is *everything*. Tozer reminds us of the biblical truth that a heart fully surrendered and actions totally submitted to God will result in real fruit.

Walking in the Spirit

The concept of walking in the Spirit can be difficult to grasp. Do I do it by pure self-discipline? Is the fruit something I produce? When we look at the apostle Paul's writing on the subject in Galatians we find that our part is small but significant. In a nutshell our part is to focus on God, surrender our personal desires and selfishness, and submit to his truths through prayer, meditation, and study of his Word. Paul writes in Galatians 5:16: "But I say, walk by the Spirit, and you will not carry out the desire of the flesh." If walking by the Spirit were an automatic response to being born again, Paul wouldn't have to tell us to do it! And if it were impossible to do, he wouldn't even exhort us to try. He reminds us of the intensity of the struggle as he continues in verse 17: "For the flesh sets its desire against the Spirit, and the Spirit against the flesh; for these are in opposition to one another, so that you may not do the things that you please."

How do we win this battle of the flesh and produce the fruit of the Spirit Paul spoke about in Galatians? Consistent with Paul's teaching, John gives us a clearer picture when he shares what Jesus told his disciples in the parable of the vine: Jesus says, "Abide in Me, and I in you. As the branch cannot bear fruit of itself unless it abides in the vine, so neither can you unless you abide in Me. I am the vine, you are the branches; he who abides in Me and I in him, he bears much fruit, for apart from Me you can do nothing" (John 15:4–5).

Abide means to stay in a given place, state, relation, or expectancy. It means to dwell, endure, remain, or stand. We all know what happens if we pull a branch off a tree: It dies; it has no life to produce fruit. In this parable, Jesus is speaking of specific spiritual fruit—all those wonderful manifestations of walking in the Spirit Paul spoke of in Galatians.

Children often ask for something that is not good for them. I remember when my oldest daughter got her first two-wheel bike for Christmas. She was so excited she could barely contain herself; she wanted to jump on it immediately and ride it down the street. The problem was she didn't know how. She didn't understand why her father thought she would fall over and get hurt. She'd seen all the other kids riding and it looked so easy. She soon discovered, after a badly scraped knee, it was a good idea to wait for Dad. As he gently held on and walked beside her, she began to get her balance. She wanted him to stay very near and paid close attention to his words of instruction on how to maneuver her new bike.

That is how it is with us every day of our life. We need to stay very close to our heavenly Father. We need to understand his words and let them give us nourishment and life. He wants us to glorify him by bearing spiritual fruit; but there are no shortcuts. There are no blessings that come ahead of abiding. If they did, we would not abide.

I believe that when we "practice the presence of God" it is almost impossible to not walk in the Spirit. And doing so produces a vibrant spiritual life. This has nothing to do with outward ministry and church attendance. It is simply an intimate relationship with God. We have now come back full circle to the "One Thing" . . . the greatest of all commandments: "Love the Lord your God with all your heart, and with all your soul, and with all your mind" (Matt. 22:37).

What do you think of when you hear the word *godliness*? I have been taught that it is equivalent to being "God-obsessed." I've been obsessed with food, with exercise, and sometimes even with accomplishing good things *for* God, but wouldn't it be great to be totally obsessed *with* God every moment of every day? That obsession would be healthy and positively life changing. Like Brother Lawrence, A. W. Tozer, and many others, *that* is our ultimate goal. To be so transformed by the truth of God's complete and powerful presence in our life that everything else is secondary. The psalmist wrote, "Delight yourself in the LORD and He will give you the desires of your heart" (Ps. 37:4). A complete delight in and for God produces

271

desires that are in sync with his will and purpose for us. What a wonderful thing.

If you want to live with purpose, ask yourself not only the "One Thing" questions but, more important, "What is my motive?" I believe these truths we've been exploring are at the core of life-changing freedom in Christ. They are the deep, spiritual principles that will make us women of purpose and equip us to leave legacies of eternal value.

Leaving a Legacy

If we would simply invest our greatest passion and energy these remaining years on the "One Thing," I believe our eulogies would read something like this:

- She was a woman who loved God with all her heart, soul, mind, and strength.
- She made a difference through loving others as herself.
- She touched our lives by sharing the "one thing" that gives life true meaning.

It has been said that to leave a legacy we need to live a legacy. I'd like to close this book with a tribute to a very special woman who has been making powerful deposits into my life for almost fifty-two years.

Growing up, I thought I had the perfect life. Sunny Southern California was the best place to live, and I had the best parents in the whole world. A glimpse into my life in the late 1950s would reveal an average, "normal" family living in a modest, middle-income home. Compared to other kids, I was really not anything special: tall, skinny, and crooked-toothed; quite average; and some years even homely. My report card reflected mostly Bs and my greatest gift was my vivid imagination. I really didn't excel at anything in particular, except one very important thing: I liked myself!

For a season in my teens and twenties, some of that sense of self-worth came crumbling down as I struggled with issues of insecurity about my body. I gave in to the lies that so many women in our culture believe. We tell ourselves that we are "less than" our friends, "less than" our co-workers, "less than" our husbands want. Simply put, we are "less than" perfect.

Fortunately, my season of doubt was relatively short-lived. As I came to know Christ in a personal way, I recaptured that sense of completeness I had as a child. Through the years, I have had the opportunity to coach women in how to balance their bodies, souls, and spirits. It has broken my heart to see that so many who know and love Christ don't like themselves.

I began wondering why I had been blessed with a sense of self-worth deep in my soul. While I knew I was no better than anyone else, I still felt significant and valuable. Why did I have this inner security, while so many other women I knew struggled?

I have come to realize that my healthy self-worth started building the day I was born. The affirming and encouraging influence of one incredible woman set me on the right path. My mom, Mary Lou Shansby, is the most genuine and content person I know. My earliest memories are of her infectious laugh, her deep connection with friends, and her passion for life. For as long as I can remember, she has believed in me, thought the best of me, and simply been there for me.

As I look back, I really didn't have the perfect life or the perfect family. What I did have were security and love. Even in seasons of failure or rebellion, Mom loved me in spite of myself. Throughout my life, she loved me with a consistent, unconditional, self-sacrificing love. As she did so, I developed a sense of self-worth that was not tied to my roles or accomplishments. It was an abiding knowledge that I had value simply because I existed. It was the kind of love God expresses to us through the sacrifice of Christ.

Not all of us are blessed to have loving and affirming parents, and even if we do, sometimes we fail to allow that love to permeate our soul. We cannot control or change the past. What we can control is how we deposit unconditional love into those around us. When we develop a deep intimacy with God as our first priority, we have a foundation that can never be shaken. Helping others develop that same foundation starts with depositing consistent love and affirmation that is not contingent on behavior or accomplishment. Then, when the rug of life is pulled out from under them by disappointment or failure, they will have a solid rock that keeps them strong and Christ-confident.

If we live the second half of our lives fully surrendered to God, we can't help but leave a powerful legacy by fully loving those people whose lives touch ours. Why not let every hot flash and mood swing become your reminder that loving God is all that really matters? Once that is done, everything else that is important will be accomplished according to his perfect purpose. As we attempt to manage this menopause phase of life with grace, let us always be mindful to put "first things first."

The heat is on. It's time to let your heart burn with passion for God!

Notes

Preface

1. Maryann Rosenthal, Ph.D., "Managing Menopause," *PURPOSE* 6, no. 4 (November/December 2003).

2. Maryann Rosenthal, Ph.D., "The Mastery of Menopause," *PURPOSE* 5, no. 4 (September 2002), 9, 11.

3. Danna Demetre, R.N., *Scale Down* (Grand Rapids: Revell, 2003).

Chapter 2: What's Wrong with This Picture?

1. Nicolas Perricone, M.D., *The Wrinkle Cure* (New York: Warner Books, 2001).

2. Jordan Rubin, *Patient Heal Thyself* (Topanga, CA: Freedom Press, 2003), 15.

Chapter 4: The "Change" That Transforms Your Life

1. William Backus, *The Healing Power of the Christian Mind* (Minneapolis: Bethany, 1996), 9–10.

2. Ibid., 72.

Chapter 5: The Seasons of Our Lives

1. "Seize the Day." Copyright 1999 by Salem Music Networks, Inc., a division of Salem Communications Corporation. Lyrics by Carolyn Arends.

2. Christine Gorman and Alice Parker, "The Fires Within," *Time*, February 23, 2004, 38–46.

Chapter 6: You Go . . . Go . . . Go, Girl!

1. Dr. Richard Swenson, *Margin* (Colorado Springs: NavPress, 1992), 13.

2. T. D. Jakes, *Maximize the Moment* (New York: G. P. Putnam's Sons, 1999), 13.

Chapter 8: Exercise—Use It or Lose It!

1. Caltrac Activity Monitor is manufactured by Muscle Dynamics Fitness Network in Torrance, California, and is available at www.DannaDemetre.com.

Chapter 9: Does Menopause = Fat?

1. Life Wellness Pharmacy, Inc., Bio-Identical Hormone Replacement Therapy in Carlsbad, California. www.lifewellness.com.

Chapter 10: The ABCs of Lifestyle Change

1. Francisco Contreras, M.D., *The Hope of Living Long and Well* (Lake Mary, FL: Siloam Press/Strang Communications Company, 2000), 93.

Chapter 11: HRT—Yes or No?

1. Mark Stengler, *Your Menopause, Your Menotype* (New York: Avery, 2002), 4.

2. Ibid., 83.

3. Amanda Spake, "The Hormone Conundrum," *U.S. News & World Report* 136, no. 9 (March 15, 2004), 62.

4. Ibid., 61.

5. Ibid.

6. Stengler, *Your Menopause, Your Menotype*, 85.

Chapter 12: Hormone Hostage Husbands, Part One

1. Bill and Pam Farrel, *Marriage in the Whirlwind* (Madison, WI: InterVarsity Press, 1996), 62.

2. Ibid.

3. Stephen R. Covey, *The Seven Habits of Highly Effective People* (New York: Simon & Schuster, Inc., 1989).

4. Gary Chapman, *The Five Love Languages* (Chicago: Moody Publishers, Northfield Press, 1996).

Chapter 13: Hormone Hostage Husbands, Part Two

1. Bill and Pam Farrel, *Men Are Like Waffles—Women Are Like Spaghetti* (Eugene, OR: Harvest House, 2001), 75–76.

Chapter 14: Menopause and the Single Woman

1. Diana Twadell, "Living Single in a Married World," *PURPOSE* 1, no. 4 (Fall 1997), 5–6.

2. Luci Swindoll, *Wide My World . . . Narrow My Bed* (Portland: Multnomah Press, 1982).

Chapter 16: What's Your Wheelchair?

1. Stengler, *Your Menopause, Your Menotype*, 209.

Chapter 17: Feeling Down? Look Up!

1. Stengler, *Your Menopause, Your Menotype*, 209.

Chapter 18: Living with Purpose . . . Leaving a Legacy

1. Timothy R. Scott, Ph.D., "Come Home," *PURPOSE 5*, no. 3 (May 2002), 7–9. Dr. Scott is senior pastor of Scott Memorial Community Church in San Diego, California, and holds a Ph.D. in New Testament theology. He is also president of Declare His Presence Ministries in San Diego and host of *Perspectives*, a weekly radio show on KPRZ 1210 AM, Salem Communications. Websites: www.DHP1.com and www.declarehispresence.org.

2. Robert J. Edmonson, *The Practice of the Presence of God* (Brewster, MA: Paraclete Press, 1985), 37.

3. A. W. Tozer, *The Pursuit of God* (Camp Hill, PA: Christian Publications, 1982, 1993), 85, 87.

4. Ibid., 89–90.

Recommended Resources

Danna Demetre, R.N.
LifeStyle Dimensions
1891 Fuerte Valley Drive
El Cajon, CA 92019
(619) 444-3400
www.dannademetre.com
www.womenofpurpose.org

Speaker and author of bestselling *Scale Down: A Realistic Guide to Balancing Body, Soul, and Spirit.* Caltrac Activity Monitors, healthy self-talk tapes, Scale Down . . . Live It Up series, inspirational taped presentations, and more available on website.

Declare His Presence Ministries
Timothy R. Scott, Ph.D.
www.dhp1.com

Bill and Pam Farrel
Masterful Living
Farrel Communications
P.O. Box 1507
San Marcos, CA 92079

(800) 810-4449
www.masterfulliving.com

Marriage and relationship experts; international speakers and authors of numerous books, including bestselling *Men Are Like Waffles, Women Are Like Spaghetti.*

Health Solutions Today with host, **Danna Demetre, R.N.**
Weekly radio show on KPRZ 1210 AM
Saturdays at 10:00 a.m., Pacific time
Listen online at www.kprz.com
www.healthsolutionstoday.com

Life Wellness Pharmacy
Bio-Identical Hormone Replacement Therapy
1932 Kellogg Avenue
Carlsbad, CA 92008
(800) 210-9434
www.lifewellness.com

Mark Stengler, M.D.
La Jolla Whole Health Medical Clinic
950 Villa La Jolla Drive, Suite 1172
La Jolla, CA 92037
(858) 450-7120
www.thenaturalphysician.com

Author of several books, including *The Natural Physician's Healing Therapies*; *Your Vital Child*; and *Your Menopause, Your Menotype.*

Books

The Practice of the Presence of God by Robert J. Edmonson
(Brewster, MA: Paraclete Press, 1985).
The Pursuit of God by A. W. Tozer (Camp Hill, PA: Christian
Publications, 1982, 1993).

Danna Demetre is the Christian woman's total life coach. Author of the bestselling *Scale Down: A Realistic Guide to Balancing Body, Soul, and Spirit* and *Change Your Habits, Change Your Life*, she has great passion for encouraging women toward greater balance in all the seasons of their lives. She has combined her professional knowledge with her personal experience to become a healthy role model for women of all ages.

Danna is president of Lifestyle Dimensions, a company dedicated to helping others make healthy and lasting lifestyle changes. Her *Scale Down . . . Live It Up* video and DVD programs are springing up in churches and ministries all over the country as enthusiastic women are sharing their personal successes and facilitating programs in their communities.

She is also president of Women of Purpose, an evangelistic outreach ministry committed to encouraging women toward life-changing freedom in Christ. In addition to a busy speaking ministry, Danna produces and hosts two Christian radio shows, Perspectives and Health Solutions Today.

Danna and her husband, Lew, have three grown children and an eight-year-old adopted grandson, Jesse. They live in San Diego, California.

Danna can be reached at www.dannademetre.com

Inspiration *and* insight *for a* woman's middle years.

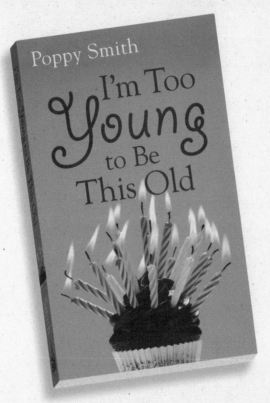

With plenty of humor, Poppy Smith leads
women through both the lighter side of midlife
and the deeper issues that concern them.

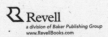